BODY ART

ARTS FOR HEALTH

Series Editor: Paul Crawford, Professor of Health Humanities, University of Nottingham, UK

The *Arts for Health* series offers a ground-breaking set of books that guide the general public, carers and healthcare providers on how different arts can help people to stay healthy or improve their health and wellbeing.

Bringing together new information and resources underpinning the health humanities (that link health and social care disciplines with the arts and humanities), the books demonstrate the ways in which the arts offer people worldwide a kind of shadow health service – a non-clinical way to maintain or improve our health and wellbeing. The books are aimed at general readers along with interested arts practitioners seeking to explore the health benefits of their work, health and social care providers and clinicians wishing to learn about the application of the arts for health, educators in arts, health and social care and organisations, carers and individuals engaged in public health or generating healthier environments. These easy-to-read, engaging short books help readers to understand the evidence about the value of arts for health and offer guidelines, case studies and resources to make use of these non-clinical routes to a better life.

Other titles in the series:

Film	Steven Schlozman
Theatre	Sydney Cheek-O'Donnell
Singing	Yoon Irons and Grenville Hancox
Reading	Philip Davis
Drawing	Curie Scott
Photography	Susan Hogan
Storytelling	Michael Wilson
Music	Eugene Beresin
Painting	Francisco Javier Saavedra-Macías, Samuel Arias-Sánchez, and Ana Rodríguez-Gómez

Video	John Quin
Magic	Richard Wiseman

Forthcoming titles:

BODY ART

BY

BRIAN BROWN
De Monfort University, UK

AND

VIRGINIA KUULEI BERNDT
Texas A&M International University, USA

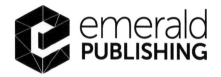

United Kingdom – North America – Japan – India
Malaysia – China

Emerald Publishing Limited
Howard House, Wagon Lane, Bingley BD16 1WA, UK

First edition 2023

Copyright © 2023 Brian Brown and Virginia Kuulei Berndt.
Published under exclusive licence by Emerald Publishing Limited.

Reprints and permissions service
Contact: www.copyright.com

British Library Cataloguing in Publication Data
A catalogue record for this book is available from the British Library

ISBN: 978-1-80455-811-9 (Print)
ISBN: 978-1-80455-808-9 (Online)
ISBN: 978-1-80455-810-2 (Epub)

Printed and bound by CPI Group (UK) Ltd, Croydon, CR0 4YY

INVESTOR IN PEOPLE

Virginia Kuulei Berndt dedicates this book to Daniel, Mom, Caroline, and Curtis. Thank you for always encouraging and inspiring me.
Brown would like to dedicate this volume to Xylia – an inspiration, support, source of gentle encouragement and constant companion on life's journey these past eighteen years. Oh, and she's the proud owner of some wicked tattoos too!

CONTENTS

ABOUT THE AUTHORS

Brian Brown is Professor of Health Communication in the Faculty of Health and Life Sciences at De Montfort University. His academic interests range across health care, philosophy, educational studies, gender studies and the health humanities. His recent projects include initiatives to use the arts to alleviate suffering and enable resilience in the face of mental health problems in both the UK and India. The core of his work has focused on the interpretation of human experience across a variety of different disciplines and settings including health and social care, education, philosophy and the arts in health, exploring how these may be understood with a view to improving practice and with regard to theoretical development in the social sciences. In particular, this concerns notions of governmentality and habitus from Foucauldian and Bourdieusian sociology, and how everyday experience reveals how systems of knowledge operate in society. He has also dabbled in community arts and been part of a group who took over derelict buildings and turned them into art galleries. Recently he has been using his spare time to plant trees in a rewilding project and hopes to live long enough to witness the forest canopy closing over his head.

Virginia Kuulei Berndt is an Assistant Professor of Sociology at Texas A&M International University in the USA. Much of Virginia's research and teaching centres on reproductive health as it relates to disasters, the environment, the body and embodiment, provider-patient interactions, and sociological theory. Virginia has presented this research in the USA, Sweden, and Canada and has published in academic journals including *Contraception, Culture,*

Health & Sexuality, Health, International Sociology, and more. In her spare time, she enjoys embroidery, browsing and obtaining tattoos, drinking coffee, and spending time with her loved ones, especially her spouse and two cats.

FOREWORD: CREATIVE PUBLIC HEALTH

The *Arts for Health* series aims to provide key information on how different arts and humanities practices can support, or even transform, health and wellbeing. Each book introduces a particular creative activity or resource and outlines its place and value in society, the evidence for its use in advancing health and wellbeing, and cases of how this works. In addition, each book provides useful links and suggestions to readers for following-up on these quick reads. We can think of this series as a kind of shadow health service – encouraging the use of the arts and humanities alongside all the other resources on offer to keep us fit and well.

Creative practices in the arts and humanities offer a fantastic, non-medical, but medically relevant way to improve the health and wellbeing of individuals, families and communities. Intuitively, we know just how important creative activities are in maintaining or recovering our best possible lives. For example, imagine that we woke up tomorrow to find that all music, books or films had to be destroyed, learn that singing, dancing or theatre had been outlawed or that galleries, museums and theatres had to close permanently; or, indeed, that every street had posters warning citizens of severe punishment for taking photographs, drawing or writing. How would we feel? What would happen to our bodies and minds? How would we survive? Unfortunately, we have seen this kind of removal of creative activities from human society before and today many people remain terribly restricted in artistic expression and consumption.

I hope that this series adds a practical resource to the public. I hope people buy these little books as gifts for family and friends, or for hard-pressed healthcare professionals, to encourage them to revisit or to consider a creative path to living well. I hope that creative public health makes for a brighter future.

Professor Paul Crawford

1

DEFINING THE FIELD: THE MULTIPLE ARTS OF THE BODY

Body art – especially in the form of tattoos and piercings – has enjoyed an explosion of interest in many nations in the last 30 years. It is hard to estimate just how many people have taken up this trend, but some authors suggest that perhaps between 21% and 29% of Americans have a tattoo (Pittman et al., 2022) with younger adults leading the practice. However, with an activity which is growing in popularity like this, estimates quickly become outdated, so any figures quoted are only the roughest of rough guides. We can say with some confidence, however, that in the nations of Europe, North America and the so-called 'Global North' (which, confusingly also includes Australasia) this kind of body art is embraced by a substantial minority of people.

It is usual to start academic texts with definitions, but in this case it's hard to know how wide to cast the definition of body art. In general, people think about tattooing and piercing under this heading, but it could potentially include much more. There is also scarification, where scars are deliberately created for ritual or decorative purposes through branding or cutting of the skin, along with implantation, where implants are inserted under the skin to create textures and contours, to name only a few of the practices which could be thought of as body art. And there's more – could body building or cosmetic surgery be thought of as kinds of body art, too? Long after their heyday in the nineteenth century, it is possible to find people in the contemporary era reducing their waists with corsets. 'Waist-training' and corseting circles are thriving communities, popularised in part by a contemporary renaissance of hourglass shapes being the ideal feminine figure and a revival of interest in retro needlecrafts. Could this be considered a kind of body art? As well as the shape or appearance of the body, there are also its capabilities. We probably wouldn't consider endurance runners to be practising a kind of body art, but if they wanted to be thought of like this, it would be hard to say no, as they train and reshape their bodies, savouring each run as an almost sacred ritual. As well as the relatively enduring kinds of body art like tattooing and piercing, there are a variety of more transient art forms jostling for attention such as body painting and henna decoration. Even with piercings, the holes may readily heal up, and some people deliberately undertake 'play piercings', which are intended to be temporary. There are also a variety of temporary tattoos to stick or transfer on for those who want a short-term decoration. In a similar vein, there is clip on jewellery that resembles the kind used in body piercing.

The areas of the body involved and the kinds of practice are changing too. On first inquiring about a tongue piercing in 1995, one of us (BB) was told that it was a well-nigh impossible and fraught with danger, and that no one managed to keep them in long before being overcome with infection. Receiving one involved a trip to a major city several hours away. Yet, nowadays these are fairly common piercings. It is a good idea to advise potential clients of the possible side effects of any body art, of course, but the sheer wall of impossibility which was thought to exist in the 1990s has now been overcome, and the procedure is much more accessible. In a similar way, in the 1990s, tattooists were reluctant to tattoo conspicuous areas like the hands and the face, yet in the 2020s, these kinds of tattoos are becoming more commonplace, and not just amongst entertainers and social media personalities either. We shall turn to the question of changing fashions and patterns of social acceptability later in considering the path of the decorated individual through the vicissitudes of family life, working life and interactions with the wider society. The point here is that everything is in a state of change, and it is therefore difficult to say anything definite about either body art or the very capabilities of the body itself.

We still have not quite answered the question of what body art involves. Turning to other writers who have addressed the question of body art, we find that they have grappled with the issue of what exactly it is they're talking about in different ways. Body art might include modifications that are non-medical and voluntary (Keagy, 2015), whereas some limit the scope to piercings and tattoos (Martin & Cairns, 2015), or focus entirely on piercings (Swami et al., 2012). Others include a greater variety of body projects that allow individuals to be and display their true selves: life-changing and life-saving measures including medically mediated procedures like gender affirmation (Aguayo-Romero et al., 2015), weight loss or gain and even cosmetic surgery (Karupiah, 2013). These procedures help to 'achieve permanent alterations of the human body' (Stirn et al., 2011, p. 359). Some authors focus on people with more unusual, extensive or conspicuous modifications (Atkinson & Young, 2001; Klesse, 1999). David Lane (2017), in a wide-ranging review of the different ways in which body art and body modification has been defined and studied, offers four features that run through most of the activities that are subsumed under this heading. First, body art modifications are performed for aesthetic reasons, rather than, for example, medical benefits. Second, they alter the organic form of the body for a period of time. Third, they are intended for at least one person – including the wearer – to see. Fourth, they are considered to be part of the cultural sphere of body modification (Lane, 2017, p. 3). This fourth point can be rather elastic – body modifications can be whatever body modifiers consider them to be. So, we get only a little closer to any precision! However, the discussion so far might give some idea of the activities that can be called 'body art' or 'body modification'.

Following on from this, it would seem that the opportunities for engagement with body decoration as a spectator appear to be rather extensive. It is widely depicted in a variety of forms of media. There are a great many social media accounts whose owners show off their body art collections, and it forms an important part of the legacy media too, providing a subject for documentary and magazine programme makers, or merely providing a colourful backdrop via characters' piercings and tattoos. Sometimes they are a specific focus of the story – films with titles like 'The Girl with the Dragon Tattoo' give some hint as to the contents! On other occasions, the decoration is more incidental to the plot yet lends a more exotic and visually arresting feel to the *mise-en-scene*. Once upon a time, perhaps less than 30 years ago, seeing body art in the media needed a trip to the shops to get one of a handful of tattoo magazines, which in the United Kingdom at least, were not widely stocked. Yet, now it appears to be everywhere and is consumed ceaselessly, through scrolling and 'binging' television shows like *Best Ink, Ink Master, Tattoo Redo, Miami Ink, LA Ink* and more.

Before we go any further, to head off another source of confusion that we might encounter when reading around the subject, it is worth bearing in mind that the term, 'body art', has not always been used to denote such things as tattoos, piercings and allied manipulations of the body. From around 1960 to the late 1980s, the term referred to works of art which incorporated the 'artist's body ... rather than the more conventional wood, stone or paint on canvas' (Atkins, 1991, p. 73). This might include, for example, the work of Yves Klein who had his naked female assistants smear blue paint on canvases with their bodies. This kind of activity was considered very *avante garde* in the late 1950s. Applying the term body art to tattoos and piercings was consolidated by the UK-based magazine, *Body Art*, which ran from 1988 to 1997. One of us (BB) actually received a phone call from one of the editors in 1997 – BB's initial pleasure at being contacted was tinged with sadness because the purpose of the call was to tell him that they would not be printing the magazine any longer and ask him if he wanted his subscription money back. Nevertheless, there was much more coverage to come in the future, from magazines to material in mainstream popular media, to the proliferation of ideas, images and stories on the internet, as the practices gained in popularity and became even more popular as a way of decorating and garnering interest on stage, screen and social media.

In the United States, the contemporary era of body art and body modification was ushered in by such pioneers as Richard Simonton (better known by his pen name, Doug Malloy), Jim Ward, proprietor of the Gauntlet piercing shop and Roland Loomis (who performed under his stage name, Fakir Musafar). We will return to these early luminaries later as they were important in shaping the styles, subcultures and stories around body art in North America.

That's a little recent history behind the current movement. There are many examples which take the history of body modification much further back, of course. One of these is the so-called 'ice man', Otzi, a Bronze Age man whose remains were discovered in the Italian Alps in 1991. Having been embedded in the snow for thousands of years, the body was remarkably well preserved and has been the source of many clues about life 5,300 years ago when the unfortunate traveller is believed to have succumbed to the cold weather or perhaps to an arrow wound in his shoulder. Amongst the features of interest was the fact that he was sporting a great many tattoos when he died. Many of these took the form of dotted lines, which appeared to have been made by piercing the skin and then applying charcoal. To complement his tattoos, Otzi also appeared to have stretched ear piercings, perhaps around 7–11mm across (Samadelli et al., 2015). As archaeologists and historians have turned their attention to the antecedents of contemporary body art, many other examples have come to light. Earrings requiring pierced ears have been found as grave goods in the ancient city of Ur, from around 4,500 years ago (Hesse, 2007). Historical references to nose piercing have been found in the Vedas before becoming more popular in India in the sixteenth century (De Mello, 2007), and in the Old Testament Bible where Abraham's servant gives Rebecca a nose ring.

Like many kinds of history, of course, there is a plethora of stories, some of which are hard to validate. Many of these can be traced to the long out-of-print pamphlet by Doug Malloy, *Body & Genital Piercing in Brief*. Here, we can find a variety of anecdotes that persist into the present day, such as the story that Queen Victoria's consort Prince Albert had the eponymous piercing in his urethra to secure his manhood so it would not be visible through his trousers. Other stories that seem to be Doug Malloy-isms include the idea that Roman soldiers had nipple piercings so as to secure their cloaks, or that navel piercings were common in ancient Egypt. There is little concrete evidence to support many of these ideas.

Moreover, it would not usually be considered a good idea nowadays to use intimate piercings as loadbearing attachment points (save for brief, short-term intimate play, but that, as they say, is a story for another day). What is interesting here is not so much the literal truth of the histories which have been elaborated, but rather the fact that people thought they needed them in the first place. There was something very attractive about the idea that body art was part of a venerable historical tradition, so the histories were added, almost as an artificial patina. As Hobsbawm and Ranger (1983) have described, this isn't unique to body art. The identities of nation states, artistic traditions and folktales which are re-told for tourists are all examples of this creativity where history and tradition are concerned. The idea of Wales as a country with a tradition of music and literature stretching back millennia or Scotland as being about tartan, kilts and Robbie Burns's poetry are examples of this elaboration and embellishment of supposed traditions by folklorists and nationalists in the nineteenth century. The idea of an illustrious history is an attractive one in many fields of human endeavour, even if it eventually turns out to be a modern invention.

In fairness to Malloy and his history making, back in the 1970s, there was little to go on. In the present, with libraries of information available via the internet, it is hard to imagine the relatively restricted media environment of the 1970s and 1980s. With a mere handful of TV channels, a similar number of newspapers and histories of body art being far beyond the reach of small provincial public libraries, there was little hope of validating such stories. Conversely, it was just as hard to refute them, so once seeded into the cultural fabric, there were no natural predators for these tales as they passed from person to person by word of mouth and photocopied fanzines. Unimpeded by the present-day armies of so-called 'fact checkers' and 'disinformation correspondents' these stories flourished. Malloy's talent lay as a storyteller rather than as an empirically meticulous historian.

Another long-standing stalwart of the body modification scene in the United States, Elayne Angel (formerly Elayne Binnie) has produced a book called the *Piercing Bible* (Angel, 2009; Angel & Saunders, 2021) which contains not only practical information about technique, feasibility and safety, but also a variety of historical information which is rather better regarded than Doug Malloy's initial efforts at providing a history for the field. However, the overall theme remains significant – the need for a sense of history. Whether it can be backed up by the documentary or archaeological record is somewhat debatable, but people love these kinds of histories, both creating them and retelling the tales as if they were privy to some sort of hidden knowledge.

Despite this growth in popularity, the meanings of these practices grouped under the broad heading of body art have yet to be fully established. This book is part of a series in the health humanities, so part of our task is to consider body art as a creative and artistic endeavour and explore its relationship to health and wellbeing. This highlights another thorny area because body art has not always been well regarded by professionals and decision makers, so making an argument for its benefits can be an uphill struggle. The response to the phenomenon on the part of many health professionals and researchers has often been negative, and body art has historically been identified as a risk factor for problems ranging from mental ill health to offending behaviour. The enduring and painful quality of many body modification practices, allied to social prejudices against them, have made a variety of professional groups including psychiatrists and other doctors, psychologists and lawyers to take visible body modifications amongst their clients as a sign of mental ill health, deviance, antisocial behaviour or that they are criminally inclined (Stirn & Hinz, 2008).

Looking at the academic literature, it is also possible to detect other strands of negativity. Often, where health professionals consider body art, the overarching theme is one of risk, injury and illness. The tales of infected piercings and allergic reactions to tattoo pigments which have proliferated in the healthcare literature make it seem as if it is hard to survive the process without a period of hospitalisation. Yet, everyday experience tells a somewhat less lurid story. For example, there are a whole variety of outdoor activities, from playing Rugby, to horse-riding, gardening and mountain climbing, which confer an element of risk and the likelihood of minor (or sometimes major) injury. Yet, these risks are considered acceptable and legitimate both by the people doing the activities and the health professionals who are occasionally called upon to treat them. The vast majority of the time these activities, whilst sometimes physically demanding and even briefly painful, are widely practised and enjoyed. The same can be said of body art. Whilst much is made of the possibility of adverse outcomes by health professionals and researchers, the everyday experience, at least as far as health is concerned, is much more mundane. The intervention may hurt briefly and remain tender for a whilst but the aftermath is usually easy to accommodate and work around. Whilst tales of disaster and hospitalisation are often re-told amongst young adults, often with some enjoyment, these events are mercifully rare.

In this chapter, we have attempted to define, and explore how others have defined body art. We have noted that this is not easy, as it may encompass such a variety of practices. We have begun to hint at how academic researchers and healthcare practitioners have looked at this field in the past, in ways which have not always been encouraging. In many countries, tattooing and piercing are becoming increasingly widely practised, yet a good deal of academic literature is still apt to treat these practices as if they were a risk factor for some sort of personal pathology or that the person concerned is likely to be an offender or otherwise marginalised. This situation is changing – healthcare practitioners themselves are increasingly likely to sport tattoos, usually in places that can easily be covered up at work – so part of our rationale for writing this book is to offer a timely re-evaluation of the field and an acknowledgement of the role of body modification practices as a means of enhancing wellbeing, managing mood and facilitating social connectedness within friendship groups, subcultures and, nowadays, within electronically mediated communities.

Later in this book, we will continue the argument for the potential benefits of body art and for its inclusion within the field of the health humanities, but let us conclude this chapter with one further observation. Despite the negative mood around people with body art which has been cultivated by health professionals and other social commentators, it appears from research that people with body modifications may express some virtues and prosocial behaviour at greater rates than those whose bodies remain unchanged. They are more likely to perform voluntary work, vote, donate to charities, involve themselves with community organi-sations, report eating healthily, take regular exercise and main-tain their body mass index in the range believed to be healthy (Giles-Gorniak et al., 2016). So, one of the things we hope to do is draw attention to the way that body art can add to the quality and richness of the human experience and hence to wellbeing and quality of life.

2

BODY ART AND SOCIETY

In this chapter, we will consider the relationship between body art and the wider societies within which it takes place. In European and North American societies, some groups of people have a long tradition of enjoying tattoos – the subcultures of seafarers, soldiers, motorcyclists and music fans are well-known examples – but as body art has become more mainstream, these patterns of value, status and aesthetics need to be thought about in terms of wider social patterns and structures. We will begin to discuss how people make their own stories, narratives and identities in and through body art. There has been a good deal of discussion of 'social capital' in recent years – the idea that social groups and relationships are valuable and can help people gain in health, wellbeing and even material wealth. We will examine how some of these ideas can help us understand body art and its popularity in contemporary societies where factors such as tradition, religion and the social group, one was born into are perhaps less significant for many. We will argue that bodily enhancement through body art can be thought of a kind of 'bodily capital'. Rather like social capital, it can help build friendships and social relationships, help to grow people's stature on social media platforms, start conversations and otherwise grow the social profile of those involved.

In an early sociological comment on tattoos, Emile Durkheim (1915) mentioned them as 'material emblems' of 'collective sentiments', 'means by which the communion of minds can be affirmed' (pp. 264–265). For Durkheim, tattoos represented a material signal of belonging to a moral community. Jumping ahead 80 years or so, in the 1990s, sociologists started focussing on the body in significant numbers. This had been a peripheral interest in the social sciences for a whilst, but there was an explosion of interest around 30 years ago. For example, one of the early leaders of this movement, Chris Shilling (1993, p. 5) talks about the way that in contemporary societies there is

> *a tendency for the body to be seen as an entity which is in the process of becoming, part of a 'project' to be knowingly and deliberately developed by the individuals, who have become responsible for the design of their own bodies.*

This can be seen in the encouragement to invest in oneself to be a better, more employable individual, maintain one's health and reduce one's demands on public services (e.g. Brown & Baker, 2012). It can also be seen in the accumulation of body capital (e.g. Reich, 2018) where the body can be developed as an asset. It can be trained, shaped and worked upon through exercise and activities intended to monitor health. As Reich (2018) notes, in classical antiquity the ideal body was that of the warrior at the peak of his powers, whereas perhaps now the ideal body is that of the perfect consumer, worked on with beauty products and services, decorated in corporate fashion house style and engaged in socially worthwhile yet mainstream-approved activities. Exercising with a view to maintaining a supposedly healthy body mass index is legitimate, but jumping off cliffs into shallow water is frowned upon. In Reich's (2018) view, the practice of body art has much in common with the process of investing in the body. In that respect it can be thought of as a kind of bodily capital, accumulated through labour, time and money in a similar way to other cosmetic activities. We will return to this notion of bodily capital in a short while and explain it more fully. But for now, Reich (2018) acknowledges that there may be some communities where body art is especially valued and appreciated, in a way which is at odds with mainstream aesthetics. Equally, in a society where anything up to half of young adults are sporting some sort of body art, it is clearly no longer a niche activity.

Thinking about the nature of modern societies, one very popular idea, which underlies a lot of thinking about the rising interest in body art, concerns the idea that the former moorings of self and identity have eroded and traditional pathways to adult identity have become less stable, so they no longer offer opportunities to anchor young people's sense of self (Giddens, 1991). In this view, in modern societies, the person's identity and life are shaped less by tradition and more by the variety of contexts in which they are involved. This idea is sometimes referred to as 'detraditionaliation'. To explain this, let us think for a moment about tradition, a familiar term, defined for social scientists by Edward Shils as '... anything which is handed down from the past to the present ...'. Shils (1981) includes not only beliefs and ideas, but also objects, practices, images and institutions (p. 12). If we imagine a hypothetical 'traditional' community, we might find people guided by faith and custom, or what their forebears had done. Following on from this, Heelas (1996, p. 6) explains detraditionalisation as follows:

> *The best way to emphasise detraditionalization is to posit a comprehensively tradition-dominated past, a comprehensively post-traditional present/future, and to attend solely to the processes which serve to detraditionalize. In contrast, the best way to criticise the radical thesis is to argue that the traditional is not as traditional as might be supposed, that the modern/post-modern is not as detraditionalized as might be claimed and that detraditionalizing processes do not occur in isolation from other processes, namely those to do with tradition-maintenance and the construction – or reconstruction – of traditional forms of life.*

From Heelas's point of view then, the idea that we have become completely detraditionalised, which he calls the radical thesis, is rather overstated and perhaps instead it is possible to see an interplay between different elements of tradition being constructed and reconstructed at the same time as detraditionalisation is happening. Whichever view we take, there's a sense that these things are up for grabs, that people are deciding which bits of tradition they want to preserve and reconstruct and what they might want to abandon. So, on the understanding that the role of tradition in modern life has shrunk somewhat, the stage is set for people to develop themselves and their bodies as personal projects, as Shilling (1993) described. The argument goes that in detraditionalised communities people are faced with a need to negotiate their identity in relation to novel and often complex material conditions and in doing so they may draw on both traditional and detraditionalised values and opportunities (McNay, 1999). Hence, there may be fewer opportunities for life course waymarking ceremonies so people might draw on the 'traditional' desire for ritual, but make it out of a rather less traditional (at least in Europe and North America) piece of body art. As DeMello (2000) put it:

> *Tattooing has become for many a vision quest; an identity quest; an initiation ritual; a self-naming ritual; an act of magic; a spiritual healing; a connection to the God or Goddess, the Great Mother, or the Wild Man. For members of the tattoo community who see their tattoos as connecting them to ancient or primitive cultures, the reality of those cultures is not important. Rather it is an idealized version of primitive cultures – considered closer to nature, in harmony with the spiritual realm, egalitarian, nonrepressive – that provides the appropriate image. (p. 176)*

Reading the material that's been written about detraditionalisation, modernity and the human condition under 'late capitalism', 'advanced liberalism' and the various other terms social theorists use to describe contemporary societies, one could easily get the impression that everyday life in the global north is a complete free for all, where people make their own value and meaning. Hence, the nostalgic harking back to supposedly 'primitive' times as a way of marking one's place in the world. However, a moment's reflection suggests that this is probably a little too simple. There are still plenty of tacit rules about what you can and can't do, as well as many explicit ones. People mark off their life stages, transitions and significant birthdays and anniversaries, and the social media environment inhabited by young adults is morally and emotionally complex in ways so nuanced that it's hard for an outsider even to begin to describe. Governments continue to enact policy and pass legislation governing human conduct, and theorists of the surveillance society and the database state (Rudschies, 2022) have pointed to the increased opportunities for investigative and regulatory reach into people's lives. So maybe life is not being lived without rules nor is as easily re-negotiated as some have suggested in 'liquid modernity' (Baumann, 2000). Rather uncharitably, you could say that maybe it only looks so liquid and detraditionalised from the point of view of elderly social theorists, who have seen life change a good deal in their lifetimes and can't really understand what their kids (or grandchildren) get up to. There are still a lot of rules and ceremonies about!

Indeed, the idea that contemporary life has somehow lost its rites of passage or life course way markers, especially in present-day North American Society strikes one of us (BB) as a little hard to swallow. On the face of it, there seem to be so many – graduations from virtually every year at school, community and church events, high school proms (now aped in many parts of the United Kingdom instead of what used to be called a 'school disco'), graduations from college, passing out from military training, the celebration of legally significant birthdays and much more. This was first pointed out in old research by Roger Barker and his associates (e.g. Barker, 1968) comparing the lives of children and young people in the American Midwest with those of a similar community in Yorkshire in the United Kingdom. Compared to the United Kingdom, there were a great many more opportunities for US young people to engage in community life, and far more of what Barker termed 'behavior settings' in which they were welcomed – even expected – and the stages in their life trajectories demarcated and celebrated.

So perhaps it's not the *lack* of rites of passage that make this explanation a popular one for body art and modification. Instead, maybe it is because there are so many, it means that thinking about our life stories in terms of rituals, rites of passage and threshold crossings is an explanation which is 'ready-to-hand' as the phenomenologists would say. Thus it is not surprising that when people talk about their body art, especially where this has been done in company with others, they ascribe some sort of meaning – a birthday, a relationship, a significant life moment and so on. Yes, body art may have a good deal of personal significance, but ascribing its meaning in this way also reflects our immersion in a wider culture or map of meaning.

So where does all this leave body modification and body art? Although we have not abandoned social mores and structures entirely, it seems that there is considerably more freedom for people to do these kinds of things nowadays. Perhaps also these social changes have ushered in a new era where the body and the self are something that you develop and invest in. This may include the usual features, such as being healthy, giving up smoking, exercising and maintaining your frame within the expert approved limits of a 'healthy weight'. But investing in oneself may also include the more decorative and exuberant aspects of selfhood too, such as body art. As veteran writer on the study of the body Victoria Pitts (2003, p. 17) has argued, the body is often now treated as a 'limitless frontier of exploration and invention'. Perhaps then body art is a kind of socially transformative work. Later, in Chapter 4, we will consider the possible therapeutic or health promoting – or as it is sometimes called, 'eudamonic' – aspects of body art, but for now it is worth noting that there is nowadays some discussion of the therapeutic qualities of tattoo, which is beginning to appear in the art therapy literature. For example, it can be seen in terms of accomplishments and strengths as well as part of a process of healing. These emerging tendencies indicate a possible synthesis between body art and art therapy given that tattoos can function as a vehicle for promoting healing and exploring self-identity, as well as a starting point for clients to share the narratives of their tattoos as part of a therapeutic process. For example, in medical contexts, Roggenkamp et al. (2017) advocate

> *exploration of the personal meaning of skin art and self-identity. We suggest that as a kind of augmentation of the physical exam, looking at and talking to patients about their tattoos can provide a valuable window into the psyche. (p. 148)*

The idea of capital as something other than economic resources is often traced to the French sociologist Pierre Bourdieu (1930–2002), who famously asserted that as well as economic capital there was social, cultural and economic capital. Chris Shilling

(1991, p. 654) says physical capital is 'a social formation of bodies through sport, leisure and other activities'. Following in this vein, the notion of body capital is defined by Antonietti and Garrett (2012) as involving the individual's capabilities to manoeuvre in the field of bodily activity, informed by 'personal characteristics of body functions and socially constructed external opinions and attitudes toward' those abilities or disabilities. Bergland et al. (2018, p. 5) consider that the work to create body capital may involve (1) building body capital for independence, (2) building body capital to maintain vitality and being in control and (3) building resources for social interaction.

Whilst Bourdieu's (1978) work on the sociology of non-economic capital does not primarily focus on the body, he wrote about 'physical capital', and this term appears interchangeably with 'bodily capital' (Bourdieu, 1984) and 'embodied cultural capital' (Bourdieu, 1986). This includes embodied capabilities, which might include aesthetic qualities or aspects of physical comportment, that enable the individual to gain social standing within a particular social field (Crossley, 2001). These aspects of bodily capital therefore have a kind of exchange value, so they 'function precisely as capital' (Crossley, 2001, p. 107). This 'physical capital' or bodily capital, then, serves almost like a currency that can be used to help build social networks and social support, gain status and various other rewards and resources (Crossley, 2001; Howson, 2004). We often think of adornment in the form of objectified cultural capital. The accessories we adorn ourselves with are often objects with meaning, history and labour behind them – yet they are objects we can remove at the end of the day. Even though body art could be considered adornment, it falls more into the category of embodied cultural capital. It is much more physically embodied than, say, wearing the newest fashion or carrying an expensive designer handbag.

Bodily capital facilitates particular kinds of social performances. This has often been mentioned with regard to sports people. Perhaps following Bourdieu's disciple, Loïc Wacquant (2014), boxers have featured quite prominently in this literature. Personal trainers too are likely to be more successful if they match the current bodily aesthetics of fitness (Hutson, 2013). As Hutson goes on to remark, according to his participants, physical reserves can be an asset in other walks of life such as being a public speaker and presenter.

Where body art is concerned, some kinds of performance may be more difficult, for example, with more socially conservative relatives or senior colleagues at work. Yet even these can involve satisfactions and pleasures. Having undertaken the body modification in question and successfully healed it, having fought for acceptance or having witnessed the change to a more favourable social climate can all be thought of as what therapists sometimes refer to as 'mastery experiences'.

Bodily capital where appearance and aesthetics are concerned is not entirely straightforward. As Neveu (2018) reminds us, if something looks overly sexualised or too vain or mannered, it can work against the individual who is judged in this way. So, even amongst audiences who might be favourably disposed to body art the possibility of negative judgement is never entirely absent. People whose body art exhibits a high level of technical proficiency may look down on those whose tattoos look a little too home-made, for example. Moreover, the capital exhibited by the decorated person is often a relational or collective phenomenon. As Kukkonen (2021) remarks, the benefits of bodily capital do not necessarily just benefit the person with the body in question. One of us (BB), when younger sometimes found himself borrowed as a kind of novelty friend to add interest to social gatherings, and even now is approached for 'selfies' by strangers, or students doing projects for photography courses. Indeed, VKB's friends and acquaintances often use her body art as an opportunity to express openness and curiosity in ways they might not have been able to do so previously, especially in the predominantly conservative region of the American northeast where she is from. In fact, it is often VKB's more conservative, eldest relations that express the most interest in her artwork and tattoos, showing interest in the stories behind them. The decorated body itself thus becomes a means of pleasurable aesthetic consumption that is not always possible in hegemonic contexts. Kukkonen (2021) notes that this kind of bodily or aesthetic capital is often highly particular to specific settings or communities. Things that might be desirable in one place or time are less so in others. Body decorations which might be valued in one group of friends or subculture might be less well appreciated in a workplace setting.

In any event, the practices of body art may usefully be seen as a kind of 'bodily capital' – people may be undertaking the labour of decorating or changing their bodies as a way of gaining something, whether this is the admiration of their friends, garnering attention on social media, facilitating expression, giving a sense of meaning and purpose or building social bonds. Rather than being a kind of risk factor for other problems, body art can also open up new sources of community, sociality and bodily aesthetics. In starting conversations and building affiliations, body art can be thought of as a means of creating a 'strategic intimacy' (Mears, 2015). That is not to say that everyone with body decorations is doing so just to manipulate others into liking them, but rather it may be something that oils the wheels of social life.

3

BODY ART, AESTHETIC COMMUNITIES, CULTURE AND POWER

In this chapter, we move on to consider the attractions of body art in relation to wider debates about culture, community, diversity and inclusion. In the past, many authors have sought to understand the popularity of body art within particular subcultures and communities of practice. Ethnographers and cultural anthropologists have detailed, for example, the activities of the body modification scene on the west coast of the United States, amongst bikers, heavy metal music fans, punk rockers and other 'alternative' groups of young adults. These kinds of groups are communities of practice where having conspicuous body art could be seen as a way of acquiring social value, starting dialogues, building friendships and asserting identities.

In recent years, however, the appeal of body art, and the number of people indulging is now far greater, to the point where these activities could be considered 'mainstream'. So, the idea of appealing to a small group of friends in a specific subculture is perhaps less significant, and the practices and aesthetics reflect far broader cultural patterns and tastes. Indeed, the desire to prominently display this body art for the entire world to see, through social media, is increasingly common. With this broadening of the practice comes a number of intriguing and sensitive questions about power and culture.

In this chapter, we will address this via two examples which draw on debates in academic literature and popular media. First, we will consider the positioning of young women in relation to body art by means of some recent strands in feminist thinking, particularly scholarship around the idea of 'respectability'. This is apposite as it gives us a lens through which to consider how people navigate the lingering stigma attached to body art, and how they can present themselves as worthy individuals and achieve recognition in interpersonal and occupational contexts. Our second topic in this chapter concerns the sharing or exchange of body decorative practices between cultures. This is a potentially contentious topic in the light of contemporary concerns about cultural appropriation. On social media, this idea has been a prominent feature of debates about the borrowing of styles between different cultural groups, namely the tenuous line between appreciation and co-optation. Body art may be vulnerable to similar criticisms, and we shall devote some attention to the so-called 'modern primitive' movement to explore these questions.

Drawing upon feminist theory, we might ask whether the popularity of tattoos amongst young women simply reflects the heteronormative association between women and appearance, or whether it can challenge or repurpose the expectations surrounding gender roles. Whilst body art is clearly popular amongst young adults, this same younger generation is increasingly reflecting upon and campaigning on these issues. It is therefore important to examine how this intersects with how the cultural politics of body modification is playing out in the early twenty-first century.

In thinking about body art and gender, let us relate it to some of the thinking about women's experiences of inequality. Historically, where body art is concerned, women have suffered disproportionately from the stigma attached to body decoration, such that the decorated person is seen as somehow deviant or lacking in 'respectability'. This tension between aesthetic enhancement and appearing to be part of a disparaged social group is perhaps particularly acute for those who present as female. To help us make sense of what is happening here, let us examine the work of sociologist Bev Skeggs (1997) and her exposition of the idea of 'respectability'.

Skeggs lucidly and sometimes movingly describes the continual attempts of her research participants to gain status and capital in an atmosphere of judgement. Prompted by a long-term involvement with young women undertaking health and social care courses in a college, in a town in northern England, Skeggs was struck by the way they seemed to negotiate their way through the obstacles of working-class life and finding an identity through the idea of 'respectability'. It was the 'unswerving commitment' of the women to 'respectability' that motivated the author to find out why it was such an issue (Skeggs, 1997, p. 160).

As the young women Skeggs studied were doing things that wider society approved of and thought were appropriate for young women, this was a route to becoming 'respectable'. Learning to care for people – babies, children, people with health problems – was seen as a worthwhile thing to do. It fit in with familiar aspects of women's ascribed gender expectations, could lead eventually to a job as a nurse perhaps, and was felt to be of practical value, more so than what they called the 'useless subjects' offered by the college. Aside from one's studies, respectability involved pursuing an existence on the knife edge between looking stylish or looking too 'tarty'. Skeggs described her participants carefully negotiating the fashions of the 1980s and 1990s with a variety of self-imposed rules that helped to define the boundary between attractiveness on one hand and being too sexy on the other. For example, not wearing high heels with jeans, or not wearing white stilettos (a popular footwear item with young women in 1980s Britain) with a mini skirt (Skeggs, 1997, pp. 163–164). Moreover, the young women had many conversations with each other in which they criticised other women who were perceived to be violating the rules or alternatively, not trying hard enough.

These observations led Skeggs to trace the history of the idea of respectability as a way of managing the working class in the nineteenth century. The problem of how to tackle the potentially unruly, if not revolutionary, labouring classes was managed through a variety of strategies, not least of which was the cultivation of respectability. Women were identified as one of the key vectors through which this idea could be spread. Men were somehow incorrigible, influenced by the solidarities of the factory and the tavern, but women were more readily recruited to an idealised, caring, selfless and of course 'respectable' femininity.

This kind of analysis, say Dann and Callaghan (2019), can be applied to many of the tattoos sported by women. Being a woman with tattoos can open one up to a variety of adverse judgements. Indeed, the atmosphere of respectability pervades images of womanhood such that more exuberant adornments whether in terms of clothes, makeup, hair or latterly tattoos, have been looked down upon as signifying the wearer is somehow lower class or sexually unrestrained. Consequently, in Dann and Callaghan's (2019) work, they note, where women have tattoos, they are often described in terms of meaning, being infused with personal narratives – of family, community, of belonging. These kinds of stories fit neatly with widespread gendered discourses of care and of belonging. These correspond to what Carol Gilligan (1977) has described as the 'ethic of care' in the female gender role. Hence, women are able to present their tattoos as feminine and 'appropriate'. Thus, women in Dann and Callaghan's (2019) work can position themselves safely and respectably within the dominant narrative of being a caring and loyal family member. At the same time, this familial meaningfulness has its limits. It was considered inappropriate to have actual names of loved ones in one's tattoo. This had unfortunate connotations of ownership or gang affiliation, so the preferred connection with family or community was often pictorial, symbolic or allusive.

We will be returning to the nature of meaning, gender and social power in relation to body art in the next chapter. For the moment, it is worth noting that for the decorated individual, perhaps especially women, the decoration places one amidst a complex web of actual or potential judgement. For thinkers like Skeggs, this is seen to be particularly acute for people of modest means. Being working class and at the same time striving for respectability and career opportunities in caring roles one needs to be particularly mindful of the judgement of one's peers as well as the world of gatekeepers such as college admissions tutors and job interviewers. Therefore, the participants in Skeggs's (1997) research, and those of Dann and Callaghan (2019) chose personal styles that were discreet and legible within the overarching narrative of mainstream femininity. Skeggs also highlights how the labouring classes and subordinated ethnic groups were often looked at through the lens of deviant sexuality. Thus, managing one's identity as an individual worthy of respect required a very careful path to be pursued – to indicate ones' involvement in mainstream heterosexual culture, but not to look too keen, for example.

Society is a complex system, where material hierarchies of wealth and power intersect with a variety of constantly shifting judgements relating to aesthetics, taste and the boundaries of acceptability. People in Skeggs's (1997) and Dann and Callaghan's (2019) work, however, were treating the social system as if it were somehow legible and, once mastered, could provide the person with a route to a more comfortable life, enjoying the good opinion of one's peers and employers.

In this vision of society, the middle and upper classes have a somewhat easier time. They may enjoy the ability and opportunity as a young adult to pause and dabble in bohemian or *avant garde* subcultures, to spend a year or two on travel overseas, to take risks and then resume a relatively comfortable life trajectory at a moment of their choosing. Moreover, they may be able to look forward to occupational lives that permit a degree of flexibility in working hours and locations of work and may allow a little sartorial emancipation, especially in creative fields. For those less favoured, life may be defined by strict work times and limited flexibility, chafing against a nylon uniform in company livery or perhaps reflective of one's status in a heath care organisation. More flamboyant or decorative personal displays may be hard to carry off successfully and may involve penalties such as long periods of unemployment.

The sense that tattoos had to be carefully managed and imbued with meaning also comes from a study of women in a faith-based college in the eastern United States by Morello et al. (2021). Similar to Dann and Callaghan (2019), women in Morello et al.'s study described their tattoos in terms other than mere decoration. In this study, perhaps in line with the importance of religious faith in their lives, women expressed the meaning of their tattoos through their religious beliefs and spiritual commitments. This was true even where the tattoo itself was not on the face of it a traditional religious symbol. In line with the ethic of care mentioned above, Morello's participants were apt to say their tattoos showed their spiritual commitment to ideals of social justice, a connection with one's mother, or a goddess figure that represented an alternative to the perceived patriarchal principles of mainstream divinity. Moreover, another important feature was that the tattoos were usually in places which would not impede the wearer's career. In the earlier part of the twentieth century, tattoos might have signalled group affiliation, amongst service personnel, prisoners or gangs, but increasingly in the contemporary era it is a personal or familial narrative that is preferred (Dickson et al., 2015).

Perhaps rather optimistically, Botz-Bornstein (2012) claims that tattoos on women have become socially acceptable and are not represented merely as objects of male desire. She adds an emancipatory statement to the effect that tattooed women break conventional feminine ideals such as femininity, conformity and passivity, and instead help to create a space dedicated to women's priorities in which their tattoos do not attract stigma (Botz-Bornstein, 2012, pp. 53–64).

So, is body art a re-inscription of patriarchy or a route to emancipation? Well, perhaps it is both. In the next chapter, we will describe in more detail some of the stories of reclamation, healing and reconstruction that some owners of body art describe. The enhancements to wellbeing seem sincerely expressed and, in some cases, genuinely moving. At the same time as Morello et al. (2021) point out, there is a good deal of body art which is claimed by its owners to be aligned with traditional values, femininity and religious faith. It is certainly possible to use body art to challenge assumptions, redefine beauty and break out of narrow sex role stereotypes too (Yuen Thompson, 2015). Perhaps the virtue of body art here is that it can be all these things. It is perhaps 'polysemic' – capable of bearing multiple meanings. Individuals and the aesthetic communities to which they belong imbue their chosen decorations with meaning.

Let us now turn to the second topic we promised at the beginning of this chapter – thinking about the role of body art in relation to cross-cultural issues and the longstanding fascination with 'the primitive' in anthropology and art which was found chiefly in wealthier nations in the twentieth century. As we have mentioned, some people in Europe and North America styled themselves as 'modern primitives' in the 1990s, and following this, 'tribal' tattoo designs were popular in the early twenty-first century. Nearer the present, there is a contemporary vogue for Japanese 'stick and poke' tattooing techniques, tattoos with large areas of solid black pigment and some resurgence of interest in differing ethnic and cultural styles. It could be argued then that the practice of body art enthusiasts in wealthier nations treats the foreigner as somehow exotic and 'primitive'. This way of looking at people in what are now often called 'low- and middle-income countries', or LMICs, is subject to a longstanding strand of critical scholarship.

Perhaps most famously, Edward Said (1978) wrote about what he called 'orientalism'. This described the way that in both academic writing and the arts, people from the east – the Arab world, India and North Africa in particular – were depicted in specific ways. They were often shown as exotic or alien, differences were exaggerated, Western culture was deemed to be superior and authors often resorted to cliché rather than more nuanced empirically based analysis. This tied in, Said argued, with the long history of colonialism and imperialism implemented by the Western powers. Orientalism went even deeper, because the ideas promulgated in this tradition of representing the east were themselves borrowed by intellectuals and elite groups in the Middle East as a sort of romantic vision of their own culture.

In similar vein, another landmark in this argument was set in place a decade later by Gayatri Spivak (1988). In her most famous essay, 'Can the Subaltern Speak?', she wrote about how the dominant intellectual canon in Europe and North America assumed a European point of view, and people outside this enclave were seen as somehow primitive, anonymous and mute. They had what she called a 'subaltern' status and were only very rarely if ever allowed to contribute to the discourse of policy makers and intellectuals on the global stage.

The work of Said and Spivak has sparked much debate and further scholarship, much of which is still ongoing. The take-home point, however, is that their arguments serve to trouble any representations those of us in 'the West' might have of people in LMICs, and encourage a degree of critical reflection on how our ideas and representations are informed by the position of relative wealth and power enjoyed. To valorise a particular body art practice as somehow 'primitive' or 'tribal' isn't entirely innocent, even if the person doing so intends it as a flattering observation.

We have run through these arguments to provide some background to the theme of 'primitivism' in some body art and body modification subcultures. This idea of body art as linking the bearer with something primitive has been a pervasive one. In defining the field of body art in the last 30 years or so, the book *Modern Primitives* (Vale & Juno, 1989) has an iconic status. Although over 30-years old now, it served as an introduction to body art and body modification for many readers, and was believed for many years to define the 'movement'. It is a lavishly illustrated volume of short chapters based around interviews the authors had secured with body artists and modifiers, chiefly in the United States. Just over a decade later it had, according to Nikki Sullivan 'achieved something of a cult status' (Sullivan, 2001, p. 36). It was said by Lodder (2011, p. 99) to have 'changed countless lives', having served as an *avant garde* coffee table book and conversation piece for at least a couple of decades up to that point. It is believed to have sold over half a million copies. It served to bring a rather niche group of activities and people that had been coalescing through the 1970s and 1980s out of California to a wider public. There is some discussion of whether it was indeed the first mainstream book to bring these activities and the associated worldview to public attention, with some favouring Rubin's (1988) *Marks of Civilisation* or Don Ed Hardy's (1982) *Tattootime: The new tribalism* as their preferred landmark publication. Even so, *Modern Primitives* did a good deal to cement the idea that there was a distinct subculture with a coherent ideology. A variety of authors have written about this group of people they consider to be 'modern primitives' (or as they are sometimes styled 'neo-primitives') as if they were a distinct and well-defined subculture. For example, Atkinson (2003) describes the neo-primitives are 'the most influential of the new groups of tattoo artists and enthusiasts' (p. 45). In defining who they were, the figure of Fakir Musafar (or as he was more prosaically named, Roland Loomis, 1930–2018) is often granted central importance. In his stage persona of Fakir Musafar, he was reported to have said that a 'modern primitive' is 'a nontribal person who responds to primal urges and does something with the body' (Musafar, in Vale & Juno 1989, p. 15). Notice the ideas embedded in this statement – a primal urge, as if it were something ancient, primordial and irresistible, breaking through the modern veneer of civilisation, as if it represented a form of connection with so-called 'primitive' peoples or a distant human past via decorating or altering the body.

Loomis was clearly a charismatic, articulate and influential individual and succeeded in generating interest in a variety of body modification practices which might otherwise have been thought of as too risky or painful for everyday people to emulate. His day job in advertising may well have had a degree of synergy with the persuasive case he was able to make about what he called 'body play'. In a sense similar to that of advertising, he was able to create a story about it which rendered it intelligible and presented it as if it addressed some sort of fundamental human need.

The version of 'primitive' espoused in Muzafar/Loomis's speeches and writings has drawn a good deal of criticism. For example, Rosenblatt (1997 pp. 287–288) found the version of anthropology in *Modern Primitives* to be lacking. It seemed to involve the 'whole history of Western speculation about other cultures … tossed into a blender with more than a little New Age mysticism and some contemporary sexual radicalism thrown in besides'. Rosenblatt was not the only author to be critical of how non-North American cultures were represented and appropriated in modern primitive activities, these included Klesse (2000) and Eubanks (1996). To modern day eyes, exposed to discussions of cultural appropriation, postcolonial theory and the desirability of cross-cultural sensitivity, the perspective espoused by Musafar can look exceptionally crude.

Lodder (2011) adds a slightly more sober and sceptical view concerning the very existence of a distinct modern primitive subculture with a consistent set of beliefs and practices. The people other than Loomis/Muzafar featured in the original *Modern Primitives* book include tattoo artists and counterculture figures who do not espouse the 'modern primitive' subculture story. Instead, they talk about a much more eclectic artistic style drawing on a variety of art movements in Europe, including surrealism and dada-ism, rather than a credulous and Western-centric notion of the primitive. Indeed, some of the people supposedly involved in modern primitivism such as the pioneering tattoo artist Don Ed Hardy were growing tired of the supposedly tribal associations their work had gained. Therefore, says Lodder (2011), the modern primitives were never really a coherent subculture or movement, and were an invention of Fakir Musafar and a small group of his friends.

Perhaps the idea of the primitive in *Modern Primitives* and which was espoused by Loomis/Musafar is understandable in relation to the materials available at the time. If the sense one gains of peoples outside North America is gleaned from the illustrations in mid-twentieth century *National Geographic* magazines, which he credited with developing his interests, then the stage is set for a rather crude and culturally insensitive notion of 'the primitive' which appropriates practices away from their ethnographic or spiritual context. Indeed, his name was taken from a character he read about in Ripley's *Believe it or Not* comic. At that time, the development of postcolonial perspectives was in its infancy, as was the critique of cultural imperialism or orientalism. In addition, in the mid-twentieth century, as Marianna Torgovnick (1990) documents, there was a fascination with anything 'primitive' amongst European and North American intellectuals and artists. Gallery proprietors and museum curators created exhibitions to cater to this trend, artists and popular works of anthropology by Margaret Mead and Bronislaw Malinowski described what appeared to be a simple carefree rural life on islands as if they were untainted by modernity. It is hard nowadays to grasp the extent and pervasiveness of this enthusiasm for the 'primitive' and 'savage'. But it set the tone for many of the early attempts to provide a rationale for body art and body modification.

Incidentally, the *National Geographic* magazine itself has repudiated its former representation of non-North American cultures. In a recent editorial Susan Goldberg (2018) said 'For decades our coverage was racist' and looked forward to a more sensitive, less colonialist and more participatory approach with people the magazine reported upon.

This excursion into the recent history of body art and its representation in popular and academic media is important because it helps to make sense of some of the tensions and debates that surround the practice. The claims of 'cultural appropriation' are perhaps particularly acute where the current generation of celebrities are concerned, where social media users are quick to criticise their choices of fashion and hairstyles, but there is a sense in which this opens up a more wide-ranging debate about the politics and ethics of transfer between cultures.

It would be difficult to prevent people from different cultures noticing, and then learning from and emulating one another. The now commonplace Arabic numerals widely used in mathematics throughout the world, may have originated in Egypt, or possibly northern India and found their way into Europe during a period of Islamic influence in Spain in the tenth century. Double entry bookkeeping, popularised by Medieval and Renaissance Florentine merchants, may have been learned from an older Indian system. These two examples – and there are many more – remind us that a good deal of the modern world depends on intercultural learning. The challenge is to ensure that where this takes place in the present day the relationship is one of equity rather than exploitation and mutual enrichment rather than extraction. But how might one do this as a socially and politically aware body art fan? There probably isn't an easy answer here. Fortunately, the excesses of the mid-twentieth century obsession with 'the primitive' have receded. The intriguing and sometimes lurid photographs which once appeared in *National Geographic* are now more muted and accompanied by a more appreciative backstory of the people concerned. There is still a pattern of inequality which exists between wealthier and poorer nations and between the groups of people who reside in them. At risk of sounding trite, perhaps at the most valuable stance is to approach intercultural transactions in a spirit of co-operation. This may involve appreciating the story behind the aesthetic practices of different lands, rather than simply taking them as some sort of exotic motif, a point upon which we expand in our chapter on engaging with body art.

In this chapter, the overriding theme we have pursued is that body art does not take place in a social vacuum. There is generally some sort of real or sometimes imagined community that mediates a person's choices actions and decorations. Through looking at the work of Skeggs, Morello et al. and Dann and Callaghan, we have begun an exploration of body art and gender. These are just a few examples and we will return to the issue of gender in body art in the next chapter in more detail. The take-home message from this work is that people often tread a delicate path between individual expression and continuing to seem like a 'good person' in the judgement of their communities and families. Thus, decorations that can be narrated as representing family and faith may be popular. There is also a sense that body art can be deployed as an assertion of individuality against oppressive social conventions, perhaps particularly those associated with gender, as described by Botz-Bornstein. This latter approach is perhaps less widespread, but may be more eye catching. Even so, the story about redefining or subverting notions of femininity is an attractive one within some aesthetic communities.

Our second example, the 'modern primitive' movement, was chosen to highlight how body art and body modification take place within a broader arena of cultural politics. The celebration of 'the primitive' in the arts and in body modification circles which flourished in the twentieth century looks distinctly off-key nowadays. Contemporary concerns with cultural appropriation in popular culture and postcolonialism in academic circles mean that such borrowing at least gives pause for thought. It is hard to imagine a world where the distribution of ideas, aesthetics and technical expertise did not take place. It may be difficult to 'stay in your lane' and to do so we might need to renounce a good many civilisational gains of the last few thousand years. Equally, looking ahead it may be possible to explore cultural and aesthetic traditions in a spirit of co-operative inquiry, rather than as a way of finding artefacts to plunder.

4

THE PLEASURES OF DECORATION

Where body art is concerned, the question is often asked, 'why do people do this?' After all, there is often some pain involved, there is healing time to account for, and there may be some disadvantages to the decorated individual vis-á-vis mainstream society. We have already talked about body capital, and we have mentioned how body art links people to particular aesthetic communities and broader social structures such as culture and gender. In this chapter, we will delve a little further into possible motivations, advantages, benefits and patterns of value which make body art practices attractive.

This draws on a variety of sources, such as our own experiences, those of friends, as well as the published literature there may be a variety of possible motives, intentions and rewards associated with body decoration. Indeed, we are going to unpack the idea of motivation a little, too, as this is often a rather crude idea and often doesn't capture the rich tapestry of intentions and desires that surround body modifications and decorations. The modern primitive approach which we described in the previous chapter can easily be criticised for its rather crude characterisation of the so-called 'primitive' people, but it highlights the strong interest many people have in ritual, ceremony and life-course waymarking.

Therefore, it is no surprise that we hear a good deal about tattoos or piercings being used to celebrate life course milestones like significant birthdays or events like graduation. In the case of people recovering from illnesses such as cancer, their decorations have sometimes been described as a reclamation or celebration of the body, marking the regaining of health. A woman friend of one of us, who was undergoing cancer treatment, used the associated hair loss as an opportunity to get a tattoo of roses on her head. Whilst her hair has recovered, part of the design is just visible at the crown, and she says it reminds her of her success in overcoming illness. VKB, too, celebrated milestones of chronic illness treatment and recovery through tattoos, using them to convey newfound feelings of independence and to cover surgical scars so that she felt control over the marks embedded onto her body, controlling the ink into the skin compared to lack of control over the surgeon's scalpel. The two paeonies along VKB's left and right clavicle are meant to resemble wings, a symbol of independence at finally obtaining the hysterectomy she needed in order to cure her Adenomyosis, allowing her to function and thrive in life. She is not alone; this has been increasingly common in chronic illness communities, as we seek to challenge stigma by bringing awareness to illness rather than trying to hide it. Indeed, those with chronic illness often utilise the framework of 'The Spoon Theory' popularised by Christine Miserandino (2003) who was suffering from Lupus, to communicate about what it is like to live with chronic illness and to endure its effects whilst simply trying to function on a daily basis. It has been adopted by sufferers from Fibromyalgia, Chronic Fatigue Syndrome and other long-term, life limiting problems. In this metaphor, energy is represented by spoons, where the more 'spoons' one has, the more energy they have, and everyday activity such as getting dressed, making a meal or going shopping absorbs one's limited stock of spoons. The analogy describes how healthy and abled people have a seemingly unlimited supply of 'spoons' and a consistent amount each day, whilst people with chronic illness are in constant short supply of 'spoons' and will never know how many they might have each day. Hence, many 'spoonies', or people with chronic illnesses and disabilities, have taken to getting tattoos depicting spoons, sometimes alongside coloured ribbons, flowers, butterflies, or other components representing their specific illness and/or disability. The spoon tattoo is instantly recognisable as a sign of belonging within or support for chronically ill and disabled communities and can help those feel empowerment at embracing this part of their iden-tity with pride rather than shame.

In the United Kingdom, at the time of writing, there is a widely broadcast advert for the Macmillan cancer charity which briefly shows a scene in which a patient got a tattoo to decorate her chest after a mastectomy, sharing the pleasure with her Macmillan can-cer support worker. This, and other examples like it, show us how body art as part of one's recovery from illness is becoming 'main-stream', if not commonplace. Health professionals and health char-ities who might once have disapproved of body art and seen it as an inappropriate way of adjusting to illness are now embracing it as part of the recovery process.

There is, thus, a sense in which body art activity can replace and reclaim the associations of illness and disability around opera-tions, cancer treatment, side effects like hair loss and other bodily changes and adds something flamboyant and of aesthetic value. In line with the ideas we outlined earlier, this could be seen as a recapitalisation of the body as well as a reclamation. If being ill represents a 'loss' of bodily capital, then getting decorated could represent a way of adding capital back in.

In a similar way, it is not unusual for people to describe pieces of body art as representing a 'reclamation' or redefinition after some sort of trauma or abuse, perhaps reasserting ownership of a part of the body after physical or sexual violence. Body art appears to be adding something over and above what can be achieved through medical or psychotherapeutic care alone, or if a crime has been com-mitted, judicial redress by itself. An example is the case of Melissa Sloan, who we will discuss in Chapter 6, who seeks to reclaim her body and autonomy with layers upon layers of tattoos, after enduring long-term sexual abuse that began in childhood at the hands of her brother. Yet the question remains as to how this connection between body art and reclamation has become established and makes sense to those who draw upon it as part of the process of recovery.

There is a whole range of ways in which human beings cre-ate landmarks in their lives. Baking cakes, dining with friends and family, having parties, attending religious ceremonies to name but a few. As body art has grown in popularity it has adopted a place amongst these. In days gone by, a frequently heard story about tattoos, for example, was that it had happened almost by accident. One had got drunk, was with a group of workmates and one thing led to another. Especially for people with a background in the armed forces, being with fellow soldiers or sailors off duty seemed to be a predictable feature of such stories. It was some sort of accidental youthful indiscretion.

Contrast this with what you find nowadays. The motivational story is often meticulously crafted. Birthdays, life transitions, recoveries from illness and other landmarks feature prominently. That is why we say that talking about 'motivation' is perhaps a little too simple. There seems to be a much richer library of ideas used these days to create an intentional assemblage. These are worth exploring in their own right, of course, but maybe they don't merely reflect the underlying 'source code' of humanity in any simple way, but instead are part of a ready-to-hand fund of stories through which we make our lives intelligible to ourselves and others.

The intentions, rationales and motivations surrounding body art have been explored in a number of studies. There may be many factors involved, including embellishment, an expression of individuality, a connection with one's personal narrative, a mark of endurance, a sign of group affiliation, a fashion statement, expressing resistance or independence, a connection with spirituality or affiliation to a personally valued culture, sexual enhancement desire/gratification, or no specific reason at all (Wohlrab et al., 2007). Motives for women seeking genital piercing cite sexual self-expression (79%), improved sexual pleasure (77%), and uniqueness (71%) as significant motivations (Kluger, 2012). Individuals seeking to undergo piercings tend to consider their decision for several months prior, and people obtaining intimate body piercings have perhaps contemplated the process even longer (Caliendo et al., 2005; Wohlrab et al., 2007).

This centrality of meaning to body modification has been asserted by many authors. DeMello (2000) describes how post-renaissance middle class people with tattoos create narratives to legitimise their body art. We should point out that by 'renaissance', she does not mean the post-medieval flourishing of art and culture in Europe, but instead is referring to the growing interest in body art in the United States in the late twentieth and early twenty-first centuries.

For DeMello (2000), part of identity narrative creation involves crafting an acceptable post-renaissance tattoo narrative which links it to a profound, and often spiritually significant, source of meaning for one's tattoo: 'My body is my journal', as a participant in Naude et al.'s (2017) study put it. This communicative aspect of tattooing is further elaborated by Leader (2016) for whom the body is a kind of 'book', which may comprise a repository of memories and be not only a site of affirmations, but the body art itself may represent a form of creative, embodied self-expression.

Meaning is presumed to be very important in body art. So much so that some authors even suggest that regrets and attempts at removal are because the person does not have a suitable personal narrative in which to incorporate the body art and attempts at removal have to do with the lack of a suitable narrative (Madfis & Arford, 2013). Tattoo regret for some people, they say, is to do with a failure to adequately engage in these narratives. People are unable to craft acceptable tattoo narratives when their tattoos lack sufficient personal or cultural meaning, but also because of what Madfis and Arford (2013, p. 552) describe as the 'inherent limitations of symbolic representation'.

The kinds of narratives people attach to the practices of body art may relate to the circumstances in which they find themselves and the cultural themes and dilemmas in which they are involved. As Morello et al. (2021) describe, young women acquiring tattoos may see this as a part of reclaiming their bodies, or emphasising their own terms and their autonomy. Their tattoos are a 'cultural tool' through which they claim their own aesthetic choices and communicate with others. Tattoos may represent particular kinds of relationships with femininity, seeking to re-inflect, subvert or resist cultural femininity norms (Harris, 2017; Lamont et al., 2018; Yuen Thompson, 2015). Tattooing can represent an attempt to 'retrieve the female body from the oppressive gaze' (Dann et al., 2016, p. 44).

Returning for a moment to the idea of reclamation, this was once again foregrounded in a study by Reid De Jong (2022) in a study of women who had undergone surgery for breast cancer. Participants in her study described the process of gaining a tattoo and as enabling themselves to move beyond the sense of themselves as damaged, lacking beauty, femininity, or sexual appeal. Instead,

this was replaced by a sense of uniqueness, being special, and for-
tunate; as having a work of art that signifies beauty in a way that
goes beyond the conventional norms of feminine beauty. This kind
of reclamation narrative following illness or surgery is not unusual, perhaps especially where body art following breast cancer is
concerned (Klein, 2016). There were other aspects, too, in Reid De
Jong's (2022) study which are worth noting. Here is an extended
quote from one of her participants:

> *I was off the beaten path … I mean I just was kind of not
> caring and then you know once I had the pursuit to get
> the tattoo and I saw there was somebody out there close
> to me that actually does this, then I kept pursuing it. I got
> excited, I started to get excited about something again …
> it put me back on you know my life's path … I'm back
> on … the tattoo definitely got me back on track [and] it's
> totally me and it really did empower me. I like to use that
> word because that's how I felt because it was my choice.
> It was my choice to have it, it was my choice when she
> [tattoo artist] showed me the design to say either yay it or
> nay it; it was my choice with the colour, my choice with
> the design, my choice where it was … so to me, that gave
> me power. (Reid De Jong, 2022, p. 539)*

This quote contains some intriguing language – the 'pursuit' to get
a tattoo, the sense of feeling excited – understandable after a good
deal of dour and debilitating medical procedures. Also, notewor-
thy is the sense of being able to resume one's life-course and the
experience of having a choice about something. Of course, medical
procedures generally require informed consent, and there may be a
number of treatment options, so in a sense the patient has a 'choice'.
But what she is perhaps driving at is that this was about something
positive and adventurous about which it is possible to get excited.

Another of Reid De Jong's (2022) participants commented,

> *I love when a piece of my tattoo shows. It makes people
> go, 'oh she has a tattoo under there' and it's a little bit of
> a mystery; it's like a teaser and I feel a little bit like a bad
> ass. (p. 540)*

Especially in the United States, the term, 'bad ass', seems to occur frequently concerning body art, and Reid De Jong (2022) notes this as a regular feature in the interviews she conducted with women cancer survivors. A 'bad ass' might invoke the notion of a bad or frightening person, or someone who readily causes trouble, according to the lexicographers at Cambridge University Press or Merriam Webster. In addition, as Garber (2015) notes, it has also been adopted as what she calls a 'feminist rallying cry', as a way of endorsing a woman who is particularly strong and admirable.

It is hard to miss the parallels here with the body of scholarship which has attempted to address the appeal of crime and delinquency. Many years ago cultural theorist, Marshall McLuhan (1951) write of 'crime thrills for the law abiding' and more recently Jack Katz addressed the emotional appeal of crime in his book *The Seductions of Crime* (1988). Here, the sensual experiences and emotional states of the social actor are significant aspects of various forms of transgression. Katz is talking about the emotional seductions of crime, but the idea could equally be applied to the emotional appeal of body art. The pivotal emotional moment is the act of being 'seduced': the transgressive action (whether it be a crime or a piece of body art) develops a life of its own and exercises a particular charm, standing out from the mass of other opportunities and choices in a way which is hard to explain, it lures you ('take me'). For Katz there is a kind of complicity between the social actor and the transgressive act. The opportunity presents itself in a quasi-magical way.

We are talking about body art here, and Katz (1988) was talking about crime. But the two phenomena have some parallels. Think about Reid de Jong's (2022) participants above talking about being 'bad ass' as a result of acquiring a tattoo, or Bev Skeggs's (1997) participants navigating the unwritten rules of 'respectability' in as previous chapter. Despite all that has changed to render body art more acceptable and commonplace, there is still a sense of doing something naughty or slightly taboo, entering an exclusive band of initiates and defying the dominant social narratives of who we should be and what we should look like.

Returning for a moment to Reid De Jong's cancer survivors, we can see here the role of positive emotions in their experience of themselves and how this is tied in with the aspects of doing something unusual or a little transgressive. For example, here is a woman on her sixties taking pleasure in her appearance:

> *Since I've got my tattoo, I look at myself in the mirror every time I get out of the shower (laughing). I have a smile on my face, ear to ear. It's beautiful and it's me and its now. I'm very happy with it, it's just ah, it's just that it did change me, it really changed how I felt about myself and how I looked at myself. I'm a 65-year-old woman that got a chest tattoo after a mastectomy and I think it's beautiful. (Reid De Jong, 2022, p 540)*

This sense of pleasure in the physical self is worth pausing over and considering. There are by now several decades worth of feminist inspired writing about the often-difficult relationship women have with their bodies. Anxieties over weight and shape, eating disorders, striving to match beauty ideals and subjecting oneself to beauty procedures, exercise and diet regimens which may be onerous and painful have been well documented, but a few landmark publications in the field include *Fat is a Feminist Issue* (Orbach, 1978) *The Beauty Myth* (Wolf, 1990) and *Unbearable Weight* (Bordo, 1993) which have become classics, and many more could be added to this list. So, in the face of this litany of grief, taking pleasure in the body is not only personally refreshing, but also perhaps emancipatory at a more collective level.

This sense of talking pleasure in the body is also present in other metaphors of the benefits of body art. The notion of the body as a journal or book, for example, which we mentioned earlier also comes to the fore in the following poem by Metzger (1988, p. 71).

> *I am no longer afraid of the mirrors where I see the sign of the amazon, the one who shoots arrows. There is a fine line across my chest where a knife entered, but now a branch winds about the scar and travels from arm to heart. Green leaves cover the branch, grapes hang there, and a bird appears. What grows in me now is vital and*

does not cause me harm. I think the bird is singing.
When he finished his work, the tattooist drank a glass of
wine with me. I have relinquished some of the scar. I am
no longer ashamed to make love. Love is a battle I can
win. I have a body of a warrior who does not kill or
wound. On the book of my body, I have permanently
inscribed a tree.

There are a number of valuable points here which help identify
some of the facets of reclamation and recovery. First, the way
that, after surgery, body art is pursued not just as an end in itself,
but it occasions other activities like creative writing such as this
prose-poem. It is therefore a catalyst for other kinds of creative
expression and their associated social connections and mastery
experiences. Whilst this is mere speculation, getting one's poem
published probably gives the author some sort of boost. It is likely to be different from the experience of being a patient, at any
rate. Second, notice that there are associations with insignia of life,
strength and power. Trees growing, feeling like a mythical Amazon,
birds singing and the like, in contrast to the usual rather dire associations surrounding cancer. Third, the way the body art is said to
enable her to resume intimate life, without feeling ashamed. We
know from studies of quality of life and cancer survivorship that
romantic and intimate life can pose a stumbling block. Not solely
because of changes in one's physical capabilities either, but feeling
ashamed, feeling ugly, lacking confidence and not wanting a present or future partner to see one's post-operative body. It is easy
to imagine that these preoccupations can dampen desire. But, in
this case, the author feels re-equipped to enter into romantic and
intimate situations. Finally, running through all these observations
is the reconstruction of the self as an actor or agent rather than a
passive or abject recipient of health care – in other words, some-
body who can do things.

There is also a sense in which tattoos represent a process of
branching out on one's own, away from the medical imperatives.
The loss of breast tissue to cancer treatment can be addressed with
reconstructive surgery and prosthetic objects to be placed inside
one's bra. In her book, *The Cancer Journals,* Audre Lorde (1980)

wrote about the absurdity of feeling pressured to wear a prosthesis
after her mastectomy, remarking:

> *Yet a woman who has one breast and refuses to hide that*
> *fact behind a pathetic puff of lambswool which has no*
> *relationship nor likeness to her own breasts, a woman*
> *who is attempting to come to terms with her changed*
> *landscape and changed timetable of life and with her own*
> *body and pain and beauty and strength, that woman is*
> *seen as a threat to the 'morale' of a breast surgeon's office!*
> *(pp. 59–60)*

Lorde (1980) captures how these efforts are all about reshaping the
woman into what she's 'supposed' to look like. A response involving
body art on the other hand involves taking one's life trajectory and
personal aesthetics in a different direction, which is, perhaps, more
self-defined. Indeed, people with breast cancer sometimes elect to
have realistic nipples tattooed on their breasts following mastectomy,
a service that many tattoo artists will complete for free to support
clients' reclamation of their bodies. Of course, you don't have to
choose one or the other – some people do both. But the opportunity
to step off the Beauty Myth conveyor belt and do something different has been made more accessible through body art.

These reclamation stories of people undergoing tattoos after surgery have had other effects too. The demand for this sort of healing
or reclamation is leading to innovations in technique too. Here is
David Allen, talking about performing these tattoos in no less an
organ than the *Journal of the American Medical Association*:

> *Traditional tattooing is relatively heavy-handed, typically*
> *relying on 5 to 9 needles for drawing hard outlines, then*
> *11 or more needles to fill in the lines with solid color.*
> *Given what the women's skin has been through, I need*
> *to be more thoughtful and gentler. My technique is essen-*
> *tially pointillism, as opposed to the standard slathering*
> *of color, and is oriented toward efficiency and minimal*
> *trauma. I use a quiet, lightweight rotary machine and a*
> *small grouping of 3 needles directed toward one point.*
> *The needles and skin meet while I hold the machine and*

tube as perpendicular as possible, moving and adjusting dimensionally over the lay of the skin. My other hand stretches the skin taut during the application. It also works as a depth gauge based on variations in the vibratory response of the epidermis and papillary dermis, given its postsurgical density and elasticity. (Allen, 2017, p. 673)

This is an example of how artists themselves are leading the field, in response to interest from post-operative clients. In this respect, it is likely that they know as much about how the skin responds as any medically trained dermatologist. This then represents a democratisation of expertise too. Knowing about bodies, skins and healing processes is not confined to the ivory tower or the teaching hospital, but is found in the body artists' craft too. It may be that formal research in dermatology, rehabilitation or disability studies catches up eventually, but until then, body art can be a place where people can, for a time at least, escape the medical gaze and retrieve a sense of autonomy and dignity.

Now, before we get too carried away by the liberatory possibilities of body art or recommend it as a panacea for cancer survivors, let us sound a few notes of caution. Is body art ever going to seriously disrupt the broader impress of social power? Or to put it another way, can we tattoo ourselves out of heteropatriarchy? Well, probably not. Yes, it can make people feel better about themselves in ways which are not possible via medical treatment or psychotherapy alone. This is certainly not a trivial benefit. But it is important not to be overly optimistic about its ability to transform society. That takes a lot more dedicated and often unglamorous work of a more conventional kind – campaigning, holding meetings, lobbying politicians, fundraising, protesting and the like.

Another strand of critique comes from veteran feminist author and campaigner Sheila Jeffreys whose classic *'Body Art' and Social Status* (Jeffreys, 2000) presents a far less salubrious picture. Thinking of body art as something emancipatory or subversive, she says, is mere postmodernist sophistry. Instead, she aligns body art with practices such as self-injury, female genital mutilation and cosmetic surgery that involve oppression rather than liberation; mental ill-health rather than wellbeing. She sees these as practices that are imposed rather than freely chosen and often applied to people who are disempowered or marginalised – the young, women, people who are gay or lesbian, for example. She points in particular to the risk of young women being persuaded or coerced into undergoing body modifications by boyfriends and husbands. Consequently, for critics such as Jeffreys, body art is an extension of heteropatriarchy rather than its antithesis. Now, we probably wouldn't want to follow Jeffreys in every respect. After all, both of us have acquired a good deal of body art ourselves, and it doesn't exactly feel like some sort of badge of oppression. But just because something feels enjoyable doesn't mean it will lead to liberation. Activities, pleasures and pastimes can easily be weaponised, sometimes without our noticing.

There isn't an easy way of deciding upon a single, politically correct line to take in these kinds of debates. On a more personal level, it is possible to see aesthetic and cultural pleasures going hand in hand with challenges to inequalities. One of us (BB) has been involved in some projects examining the role of the arts and humanities in fostering resilience and combatting mental health problems in India. Two of these projects currently have websites if any readers are interested (http://www.mehelp.in/ and http://mhri-project.org/). This is not just shameless self-promotion, but rather to illustrate that even when people appear to be hemmed on all sides by material deprivations, cultural and aesthetic life doesn't disappear. Indeed, it is sometimes even more important. The value of moments of enjoyment and exuberance is all the more intense. The ability of activities such as music, performance, arts and crafts to bring people together may even lead to more substantive action, and can lead to their being able to campaign effectively for a better share of national resources. People whom we involved in community theatre activities in Pune were able to lobby successfully for adequate refuse services for their neighbourhood and those involved in our mental health literacy project in Kerala have been active in campaigning for better provision and greater understanding for people with mental health problems. What is inspiring is that these initiatives have come from people themselves, rather than being something imposed by 'Western' development workers.

These projects were not about body art, but they illustrate how cultural and aesthetic activities can enable groups of people to exercise a new-found voice and assertiveness in the larger body politic. Going back to our observations about cancer survivors, the sheer visibility of this way of tackling recovery and rehabilitation nowadays has opened up spaces for new conversations and politico-economic shifts in our response to suffering. It's not just 'doctor (or policymaker) knows best' anymore. With the diffusion and democratisation of restorative resources, this lessens the hold of major institutions and corporate interests on health and wellbeing, so it is possible for people to do more for themselves and one another. With some illnesses, such as the cancer survivors we have mentioned, in a sense the tattoo represents a transition out of the illness phase of one's life towards recovery, whereas in other cases, such as the spoons tattoos, they could be seen as a commitment to an illness identity. It is perhaps significant that these latter tattoos have gained popularity in relation to 'contested illnesses' such as Fibromyalgia and Chronic Fatigue Syndrome where there has been ambivalence amongst the medical and research communities about the nature and possible causes of the conditions. It is therefore perhaps a concrete assertion of the physicality of the problem in the face of possible scepticism.

It might be possible to skim through this chapter and gain the impression that the pleasures of body art are all mixed up with reclamation and recovery. Whilst illness, abuse and deprivation are, sadly, persistent features of the human condition, this is not the whole story. It is perfectly possible to enjoy the arts of the body without having to be a cancer survivor, for example. We have elaborated on this aspect, here, because it is a particularly notable strand in the literature. It also illustrates, in participants' own words, how the body can become an object of aesthetic pleasure, a source of feelgood emotions and even romantic interest. It invites the romance of the 'bad ass' in a relatively safe way – no risk of arrest or imprisonment! – and it facilitates a rather swashbuckling, devil-may-care demeanour, which may represent a welcome change from prolonged medical treatment or years of trying to fit into perceived societal standards which may themselves be onerous and oppressive.

5

HOW CAN I ENGAGE WITH BODY ART?

The practice of permanent and semi-permanent forms of body art has become much more widespread and accessible. With the popularity of tattooing and piercing increasing in many nations, there exist ample opportunities for acquiring such decoration. Body art establishments are now more apt to resemble health spas and aestheticians more than the stereotype of a dingy establishment in an area frequented by sailors – if indeed the latter ever existed! The diversification of the professional body art workforce and styles of work available has meant that it is more likely than ever before that the prospective client can find an artist to their liking.

One key example includes the growing acceptability and refining of scarification techniques involving branding and cutting, where a sterile environment and expertise is not just essential but vital. Once primarily a practice across the continent of Africa to signify rites of passage, identities and roles, scarification has become increasingly present in contemporary society, globally (Schildkrout, 2004). Many are now at least aware of scarification, more so since the 1990s when an infamous case of consensual branding led to the conviction of a man who branded his initials into his wife's buttocks at her request (Oultram, 2009). These days, scarification primarily takes place in controlled, sterile environments;

with branding, the process involves painstaking precision to ensure the skin is burned in a specific way, and cutting involves removing a certain depth of flesh – enough to display the design but not too deep to compromise clients' health. This process is so intricate that the risk for potential complications has led four states in the United States to prohibit it outright, along with 16 states that carefully regulate scarification (Breuner & Levine 2018). The healing process, thus, takes an enhanced degree of vigilance and maintenance than healing a tattoo or piercing, for instance. The design 'comes to life' through the way the skin heals through scarring to create raised tissue to form and display the intended design. Additionally, scarification is even more permanent than tattoos and certainly more permanent than piercings. Scars are not easily tattooed over, and they cannot be removed without also removing the skin around the scar, which would leave yet another scar in its wake. With tongue splitting, or bifurcating the tongue to creating a 'forked' appearance, one must seek an oral or plastic surgeon to minimise infection risk or damage to one's tongue.

Clearly, the human body is relatively robust and has considerable powers of recuperation in the face of injury. Whilst adequate hygiene and appropriate technique are important, it is equally important to bear in mind that in proportion to the large number of body art interventions undertaken, the number of complications requiring additional medical intervention is comparatively small and often quickly resolved, in the same way as any other small wound.

When it comes to tattoos, artists differ in their style and specialty, so it is worth examining their portfolio of activities and work completed. Thanks to social media, particularly photo-sharing applications like Instagram, it is easier than ever to view artists' entire portfolios with a glance, a scroll or a tap. Many artists also create and maintain professional websites, where potential clients can browse their portfolios and submit a form to inquire about booking an appointment.

However, with technological developments comes creative ways of swindling prospective clients. Fraud accounts of well-known artists abound on social media, as do artists who post other artists' work on their own social media profiles, where they falsely claim ownership. Some argue that artists photoshopping, filtering or otherwise altering pictures of their tattoos is a form of scamming that renders the entire tattoo 'fake' (Moss, 2021). It is therefore helpful when the client is reasonably confident that the artist has actually done the work depicted, rather than it being material that they have edited/altered or copied. For tattooing, following Instagram accounts like @tattooedtruthfairy allows viewers to view examples of filtered and photoshopped pictures of tattoos so that they can be more informed and set realistic expectations from their potential artist. Ainslie Heilich advises prospective clients to examine tattoo photos for 'black sections that are very black, with no reflection and no visible pores on the skin; and white parts that appear to glow, (quoted in Moss, 2021). Visiting the shop in person to view a physical portfolio can be reassuring, and personal recommendations from friends and acquaintances who have acquired interesting or admirable pieces of body art are valuable in making decisions about artists or designs.

In the realm of tattooing, clients now have ample agency and a wide array of skilled artists from which to choose in hopes of obtaining custom or 'flash' designs onto their bodies. It is thus understandable that clients may be especially exacting about the style, colouring and size of their tattoo(s). This is beneficial, as, when creating a custom piece, artists find it helpful when clients approach them with specific ideas and an overall vision. However, it is also important for clients to facilitate artists' creative freedom, placing trust in their artistic instinct and skills. Such creative freedom is essential for an artist to successfully complete their work and to produce their best work.

Clients may also be inclined to request a tattoo bearing the image of another artists' tattoo they found online, requesting this new artist to replicate the design. Tattoo artists generally discourage this practice, instead, recommending clients use reference images from the artists' own portfolios, photos of references (pets, faces and places) that the client has taken or any reference image that does not consist of another artist's work.

When commissioning a custom tattoo design, the artist may require a consultation to ensure their style and skills match the client's desired vision. After the client's appointment is booked, artists tend to wait until the day of the appointment to reveal the final design and stencil. This timing allows the artist to design the tattoo with minimal external interference, staving off potential requests to extensively alter the design's components, up to the day of the appointment. Indeed, artists find it difficult to complete a tattoo design with a ceaseless stream of input and critique from the client, their friends and family or even distant relations. Everyone has an opinion of art, and, in this context, it is crucial to prioritise the artist's professional vision. Also, important to the artist's creative freedom and concentration is refraining from bringing an entourage of friends and family on the day of the appointment. Bringing one friend or family member is ideal for client's support, encouragement and even safety, but an entire flock of people can be distracting both the client and the artist.

At the same time, it is important to clearly communicate any points of dissatisfaction with the tattoo design before it is tattooed on the client's body. Likewise, clients are advised to provide their input on the tattoo's placement once the stencil is placed. Expectations around artist–client interactions during the tattooing process vary by artist and location. Some artists prefer to talk whilst tattooing, whilst others require as much silence as possible to concentrate (or they might not be talkative to begin with). Some studios and shops will have music playing at a high volume, whilst solo artists may prefer no music. It is therefore advisable for the client to ask the artist directly about their preferences regarding these matters, and for the client to voice their preferences as well. Listening to music through headphones is common and is usually perfectly acceptable, as long as there is not too much bodily movement from the client (e.g. tapping to the beat and dancing in the chair) as the tattooing is happening. For neurodiverse, chronically ill and disabled clients, accessible studio and artist options are increasing, as are trauma-informed artists, which we discuss further in Chapter 7, on the wellbeing of artists.

Requesting and understanding tattoo pricing can be complicated. In fact, when one of us, VKB, got her first tattoos, she did not even ask what the price would be until the tattoos were complete, out of concern for annoying her artist! Contrary to this anecdote, it is perfectly acceptable to inquire into the price of a tattoo, piercing or other body art service. What is frowned upon and may sometimes lead to an artist declining one's request is attempting to negotiate or 'haggle' the price. It is important to remember that clients pay the artist for their expertise, skill and intensive labour, and that this fee is part of artists' income, so clients should refrain from arguing about the price. Some artists have an hourly rate, whilst others simply charge a flat 'day rate'. Knowing the total cost of your tattoo ahead of time can aid with budgeting and determining a tip or gratuity. Common in the United States, tipping consists of giving a pre-determined percentage of the total cost of goods or services to reflect good service from the professional. Whilst omnipresent in restaurants and common in hair salons, tipping your artist is less of a 'hard rule'. Tattoo artists that VKB follows on social media always emphasise that tipping is never expected but appreciated. However, it is generally courteous to tip your tattoo artist, with advised tip ranges of 10–20% of the cost of your tattoo. Whilst many artists now accept credit cards or money transfer apps as payment, some still only accept cash, and tips in cash are sometimes mandatory or at least appreciated.

Clients may be dissatisfied with a tattoo they receive due to its overall quality, artistic inaccuracies, issues with colour type or saturation, or simply due to a change in tastes. Some clients may also wish to be rid of tattoos that they associate with trauma or generally negative experiences. Whilst it is common practice for an artist to decline to add onto or finish other artists' work out of respect for their fellow artists, some artists specialise in 'cover-up' techniques to disguise the original tattoo or render it invisible. Depending on the colours, shape, size and location of the original tattoo, artists may be able to successfully cover the entire design with a new design.

'Blast over' cover-up styles have become increasingly popular, where the undesired tattoo remains in its entirety underneath an intricate design that usually consists of intricate blackwork patterns. This style of cover-up tattoos is ideal for covering up colour tattoos that cannot be easily covered with a traditional 'cover-up' design. Whether a 'blast over' or a conventional cover-up, it is essential that clients trust the artists' judgement of whether they will be able to successfully cover the tattoo; not all tattoo artists are cover-up artists. Laser tattoo removal has rapidly evolved and can become more refined in recent years. Whilst it is expensive, painful and may not be able to remove certain colours, laser tattoo removal remains an option for those who wish to remove ink from the skin.

Permanent forms of body art are not for everyone of course. There may be a whole host of reasons why people would be hesitant to modify their bodies on a long-term basis. Religious faith, concerns about the permanence of certain interventions and the desire not to upset loved ones or family members may all be considerations. In cases like these, it is perfectly possible to engage in less permanent forms of decoration. A large range of temporary and 'semi-permanent' tattoos are available in a variety of styles. Whilst the small, novelty temporary tattoos once found in cereal boxes still exist, temporary tattoo technology has evolved to 'semi-permanent' pieces that last weeks or months which not only offer temporary decoration but may represent a relatively safe way to try out an idea before committing to it. Services like 'Inkbox' feature a variety of sizes and styles that last for 1–2 weeks. Some companies, like 'Tattly', create custom designs and solicit designs from tattoo artists, themselves, offering them part of the profit from sales of their designed temporary tattoos. 'Momentary Ink' offers purported half-sleeve and full-sleeve styles that do not wrap around the limb but nevertheless cover large areas of skin, exemplifying the new possibility of trying a serious tattoo design before having it permanently inked into the skin. For more control and artistic freedom, companies like 'Easy.Ink' include 'Freehand Ink' kits with ink that can last for three weeks when applied, boasting safe and natural fruit-based ink.

Further opportunities exist with other techniques. For example, in some parts of the world henna has been used as a temporary skin dye. Elaborate and intricate henna designs are possible, and these are gaining in popularity in North America and Europe too. Indeed, the fruit-based ink that 'Freehand Ink' sells comes from Jagua fruit, originating from the Genipa Americana tree. Indigenous Amazonian populations have traditionally used Jagua for body art and medicinal remedies, but it is now available to buy wholesale from anywhere in the world, thanks to online markets, including 'Nature's Body Art'.

Like Jagua's plant-based origins, henna originates in the henna plant which, when ground into powder, is mixed to provide a long-lasting ink. Henna has been traditionally used in many cultures for many occasions and is most commonly used today in the context of weddings and religious holidays in South Asia, North Africa and the Middle East. Henna designs are elaborate and deeply meaningful due to their relationship with these events. Increasingly, henna tattooing has been available in North America and Europe, and it is even more readily available online than Jagua, meaning anyone can self-apply their own henna art.

Whilst engaging with these non-permanent forms of body art that originated in Indigenous populations and in South Asian culture, it is important to be mindful of the line between appreciation and appropriation. Appropriation manifests when these art forms are turned into quick-profit commodities diluted of their cultural meanings. A sacred tradition with deep and symbolic yet clear meaning becomes diluted into plastic-packaged, cheap, fast-fashion 'Mystical body art from the *Far East*' (Maira, 2000; emphasis theirs) and 'how-to henna' books describe henna as 'capricious, mysterious, and elusive' (Fabius, 1998, p. 32). Thus, whilst non-South Asians wearing henna appear to be 'trendy' or 'cool', South Asian women are still hegemonically perceived as 'strange' or 'exotic' 'Others' or may not be able to access/afford elaborate henna designs themselves (Maira, 2000).

This does not mean that people outside of these cultures are forbidden from participating in these art forms. Rather, as mentioned in our previous chapters, deliberately acknowledging the origins of these art forms gives due credit to and centres the marginalised cultures from which they originate, and conscious efforts to learn more about the meanings and conventional designs associated with cultures and traditions enriches one's experience with body art. For instance, viewing Jagua as a newly commodified fruit-based ink arguably erases the centuries-long history of its use, rendering invisible the meanings and practices of the body art created by many indigenous Amazonian communities. It is thus recommended to research about the origins and history of henna and Jagua, watch videos of experienced and respected artisans explaining their craft, and, if possible, obtain this body art directly from artists of such backgrounds. Perhaps then, the most suitable position is what Amy Allen (2016) has called 'epistemic humility' – the recognition that we may not always know best and the recognition of other people's knowledge culture and traditions.

Despite body art, including its newer and more complex forms, being more prevalent and lucrative amongst celebrities and the public, more extreme manifestations of body art, including facial tattoos, implants and sclera tattooing, are often portrayed in the media and framed in everyday discourse as being 'stupid', ill-informed decisions, at best, or a sign of deviance or offending, at worst. Indeed, when facial tattoos are featured in headlines and media stories, they are often accompanied by a description of the tattooed individuals' alleged crimes or personality faults. Arguably more acceptable than face tattoos, hand tattoos nonetheless remain stigmatised, known both affectionately and seriously as 'job-stoppers' by tattoo artists. 'Blackout' tattoos, where entire areas of skin, especially limbs, are covered in solid black often yield quizzical reactions of 'why?' whilst also sometimes prompting valid questions about dying the skin darker in a way that may inadvertently echo sordid histories of blackface. Images of individuals practising suspension evoke pronounced visceral reactions from spectators who express 'concern' for the suspended individuals' sanity. Headlines about eyeball tattooing emphasise the horrors of potential complications like blindness and eyeball removal, featuring pictures of individuals crying purple tears in hospital, lamenting their decision to pursue this body art. Even academic literature on facial tattoos examines the criminality and deviance of the people who wear them, often young, Black men.

Indeed, today's societal perceptions of facial tattoos, eyeball tattoos, body implants and suspension echo how society once viewed all tattoos, as something to be feared, disrespected or mocked. At the time of writing, in the early 2020s, there are a number of examples in social media and the news which bring these issues to the fore, and it is worth considering a few of these because they represent a significant pathway for the wider public to become aware of body art.

First, let us consider an early 2020s social media influencer, @thatirishtwinmum. She is well-known for her identity as a mother with facial tattoos and exemplifies how she feels discriminated against by wider society:

> *I know it's easy for people to take one look at me and go 'oh she's a criminal, she's this that and the other blah blah blah', I smile at a tattooed person in the street, they smile back. I smile at a granny and get daggers back – strange world.*

This erases the meaning drawn from these tattoos. However, we should remark in parenthesis that the stereotype of 'grannies' as being especially censorious is not always true. BB remembers an exchange with two older women in a supermarket several years ago. 'Ooh, you've got a lot of piercings', quickly followed by, 'Go on, ask him if he's got his willy pierced ha, ha ha'. In a world where isolation and loneliness are major concerns for health leaders and policymakers, these moments of banter and laughter are probably significant in creating connections between groups and across generations. This incident recalls Jenny Joseph's (1992) famous poem 'Warning' in which she says 'When I am an old woman I shall wear purple' and goes on to describe a variety of social conventions she is intending to transgress.

Going back to the coverage of people with distinctive body art in the news and on social media, let us consider Melissa Sloan who also in the early 2020s appears regularly in tabloid headlines such as 'I'm addicted to tattoos – and now I can't get a job', 'I have 800 tattoos and have been banned from the pub' and 'Mum addicted to tattoos "forced to watch her children's school play through the window"'. These articles are written with the purpose of drawing voyeuristic outrage from readers at Sloan's 'selfishness' and 'bad' decisions. What they often neglect to mention was Sloan's lifelong history of sexual abuse that motivates her to cover her body in ink. Even though this latter information might facilitate a more sympathetic reception, it still reinforces a link in popular representation between extensive body art and some sort of trauma or tragedy – as if it were something that 'normal' people wouldn't do.

These narratives also imply that tattoo artists would readily agree to tattoo faces, hands or eyeballs to facilitate clients' 'bad decisions'. In fact, many tattoo artists refuse to tattoo even the hands of clients with few tattoos or any clients who are not, themselves, tattoo artists. Moreover, the legality of placing body implants remains fuzzy. As we have described, certain types of body art remain heavily regulated or restricted. Whilst legal in the United States, bodily implants in the United Kingdom became a recent topic of debate and discourse upon the arrest of Brendan McCarthy (known as 'Dr. Evil'), a body modification specialist in Wolverhampton, who provided services like bodily implants in addition to more extreme procedures such as removal of an ear and a nipple for two of his clients, along with tongue splitting that is usually only professionally performed in oral surgical settings. Whilst his nickname might indicate otherwise, McCarthy had (and still has) a reputation of taking the utmost care of his clients, providing high-quality, skilled work and a safe and sanitary environment in which to do so (although, in inspections, some of his equipment was found to be out of date). In fact, when sentenced to 40 months in prison in 2019, supporters including his former clients were devastated and jumped to his defence in media interviews.

McCarthy's case brought to light how far margins can be shifted in the world of body art and modification before being considered 'bodily mutilation'. Sure, injecting ink into the skin or even silicone implants between layers of skin are arguably the territory of the artist, but removal of body parts is a surgical procedure. This tenuous line has led to the legality of implants in the United Kingdom remaining quite fuzzy, with one news headline aptly and comedically noting, 'Extreme body modification – the law is clear, well sort of!', referencing the fact that bodily harm and mutilation may still be legally considered assault, even when written and verbal consent is provided. All of this is to say – whilst the shape of the body art 'field' is changing, with certain forms of body art shifting from the margins closer to the centre (Bourdieu, 1997), these margins can be snapped right back into place when powers of the law and medicine intervene.

Whilst individuals with tattoos on their arms, legs and even chests meet less resistance or negative reactions than in years past, those with facial tattoos, dyed eyeballs and bifurcated tongues still face stigma. Beyond stigma, such marginalisation erases the rich history and meaning behind facial tattoos and body modifications like suspension amongst Indigenous populations. Tattooing and body modifications often hold sacred meanings within these communities. Co-opting these practices and patterns, particularly amongst white artists and clients, renders their Indigenous origins invisible, and because white faces and bodies, often with little to knowledge of cultural meanings, are featured most prominently in the media, these modifications are often framed as 'foolish' or a mistake – a far cry from the deliberate, intentional, sacredness from which the designs and practices originated.

It is customary these days to call for regulation, accreditation and training as a way of tackling problems, not just in body art but in a whole variety of human endeavours. This kind of approach tends to assume that the state is a benign actor in the social realm and that those with established positions in the legislative hierarchy are able and willing to develop and implement regulations that are sensitive, humane and appropriate for others. Whilst there may be benefits to regulation, for example where hygiene standards are concerned, there may be other aspects of legal and policy frameworks which are less helpful. Legislation is often insensitive to changing practice and standards in the field and apt to stifle innovation, promote established interests at the expense of newcomers, and be predicated on policymakers' outdated and often somewhat distanced understanding of what happens and where the hazards lie. Where legislation and policy are implemented, this often falls on local government and healthcare providers, so there are additional funds to find and personnel to deploy to ensure compliance, thus placing additional demands on already stretched public services.

This kind of approach is sometimes called the 'legislative conceit' – if policymakers and politicians decide they want to change something, then they try to pass a law about it. The hope that this will change the populace's behaviour and thinking for the better often founders on the difficulties of implementation and enforcement. In this area, it might be asking a great deal of body art enthusiasts and artists to trust politicians and government officials whose contact with the scene is minimal to make decisions on their behalf. Perhaps the solution here is for policy and legislation to be developed deliberatively, based on extensive and inclusive consultation, and be susceptible to change in the light of new techniques, opportunities and shifts in the understanding of risk.

Where tattoos are concerned, it is easy to find pictures of those that appear poorly executed, badly spelled or which are likely to impede the wearer's career opportunities in the future. Yet, it is hard to legislate for poor taste. Indeed, sometimes the more vernacular styles of yesteryear can enjoy a resurgence of interest. Equally, it is worth the prospective client thinking about what they want and how it might work on their body. Not every artist, nor everybody's skin, is well suited to portraiture for example. Piercings close to the surface of the skin might well migrate outwards. Some projected ideas may be anatomically unworkable or require major surgery. For example, a few years ago, a vogue for trying to pierce the web of flesh between the thumb and the index finger appeared to peter out because there is so much movement in that area that it is hard to 'settle' a piercing in place and enable good healing. Finding materials to make piercing jewellery has been challenging. The human body is very good at dissolving materials placed inside it. This is not surprising; after all, like most complex life forms it has to move a good many chemicals around. In a sense, we are a little like the aliens in the popular *Alien* film series, whose blood can dissolve through the hulls of spaceships. The human timescale is a little slower, but, over time, the work of human body fluids is scarcely less aggressive. Experiments with different metal compositions and non-metallic alternatives such as PTFE have yielded a variety of options to suit more people and piercing placements.

In this chapter, we have attempted to consider some of the avenues through which it is possible to engage in body art and through which body art becomes visible to the wider public. There are far more areas which we have not explored. For example, a quick search of a major online retailer reveals a proliferation of lavishly illustrated coffee table books about tattoos. An analysis of these would need to be a major critical study in its own right. In some countries, there is a thriving scene of conventions, conferences and exhibitions, which would merit more intensive and systematic study. So the picture painted here is inevitably partial. Instead, what we have tried to do with the examples so far is show the reader some critical tools with which to tackle the field. Thinking critically about how media representations are constructed, about the cultural and ethnic origins of practices and the often-sensationalistic coverage that decorated and modified individuals receive in the mass media is valuable in that it helps us become informed consumers and even participants in body art practice, should we choose to do so.

6

FROM MARGIN TO CENTRE: SHIFTING BOUNDARIES IN BODY ART

The growing popularity of body art over the last three decades has seen some shifts in the prevalence and meaning of practices which were once in a small niche, but which have become more widespread. As recently as the 1990s, many tattooists were extremely reluctant to tattoo faces and hands, and all but a small minority of piercers were reluctant to pierce tongues, warning of dire consequences of injuring so sensitive and mobile a part of the body. Some people with more unusual and distinctive body modifications work in the industry and are, in a sense, a living advertisement for their services. For example, some tattoo artists choose to have their faces tattooed to deter them from leaving the industry.

Yet such activities are now much more widely encountered – tongue piercings could be considered almost 'mainstream' and facial tattoos have moved out of the prison system into popular music and social media culture. Indeed, celebrities with face tattoos are admired and considered beautiful – something unthinkable even in the 1990s. This, in turn, has led to a rise in small facial tattoos amongst the public as well. People who do not wish to make a permanent commitment can try one of many facial tattoo filters on Instagram or Snapchat that provides them with the desired trendy and edgy appearance. The fact that these filters have been developed and are popular reflect the changing landscape of body art acceptability.

Thus, the boundaries of what is considered possible and achievable as well as aesthetically desirable have embraced activities such as tongue splitting and scarification as described in Chapter 5; suspension, or placing hooks or other implements under one's skin from which to be lifted and hung (suspended) in air; eyeball tattooing, where ink is injected into the sclera or 'whites' of the eye; blackout tattooing featuring large areas of solid black; or obtaining implants to create new contours of the body which are now, if not mainstream, at least no longer astonishing. Indeed, people can now seek and obtain such implanted objects under their skin that add bumps or spikes to their limbs, or even horns to their head. Individuals can now navigate society with horns on their head meant to evoke those of a demon, albeit with public responses in the form of fussing and murmurings, reflecting how we have grown accustomed to the presence of body modification. Indeed, stigma and discrimination persist for those who overstep the line between 'acceptable' and 'extreme' deviance as we detail below, but these new advances in technology are generally tolerated in society, despite the scattered grumbles and complaints that accompany said tolerance.

In this chapter, we will begin to make sense of how the boundaries of bodily capital may be shifting and begin to sketch out how the role of social media and online content creation is shaping and is itself informed by these trends. There appears to be a desire on the part of many exponents of body art to develop and maintain a presence in both digital media and old-fashioned 'legacy media'. Some are seeking clicks, views, likes and followers for their Instagram, YouTube or other social media profiles, perhaps with a link to a paid-for platform promising more intimate or up to date content. There are a variety of young entrepreneurs who are making their bodies their business and their wounds their work – in other words, converting the bodily capital, the accumulated labour in the tattooist's chair or on the piercer's couch into symbolic and perhaps even economic varieties. A drastic departure from the days when the *Suicide Girls* website constituted one of the only realms prioritising tattooed models, Instagram and TikTok feature inked entrepreneurs who are making their bodies their business and their wounds their work – in other words, converting their bodily capital to symbolic and even economic varieties. Using hashtags that indicate one's tattooed status (#inkedgirl, #inked and #inkedup), marketing oneself based on a collection of body art, or creating videos describing one's experience with body art and modification are all common practices now. Tattooed women and femme individuals vie each year for a chance to be Inked Magazine's 'Inked Cover Girl', encouraging their networks, ranging from family on Facebook to strangers on TikTok, to vote for them online so that they can appear on the cover of *Inked*.

For a small proportion of people, it has become possible to make a living in these online environments, where their tattoos and other forms of body art garner widespread popularity, namely large public followings which can lead to paid partnerships, where influencers receive free merchandise, services and even vacations in exchange for promotion of these goods and services. Additionally, YouTube influencers who accumulate enough subscribers even get paid per video.

We might well wonder why this kind of route through life is becoming attractive. There could be a variety of reasons involved. It offers a degree of autonomy in one's work, far more than any young adult would usually have in entry-level employment. For those with a passion for body art, it is perhaps attractive to do something based on one's enthusiasms. In a number of nations, the world of conventional work is less likely to offer attractive career options. Looked at from the point of view of a young person seeking to find a place in the world, the picture is not an attractive one. Precarious, minimally paid occupations selecting customers' orders in an online retailer's warehouse, delivering groceries, making sandwiches, serving in restaurants or bars may be tolerable for a short while as a holiday job, but are less attractive as a lifetime career. Meanwhile, the proliferation of 'internships' has helped normalise the idea that one should work for nothing. At the same time, the price of property has accelerated far beyond the means of those on low (or even average) wages so the lure of 'home ownership' which was held out to previous generations as something that might be achieved in adulthood is looking increasingly unlikely. Moreover, this unappetising vista is difficult to avoid through conventional means. In days gone by, getting educational qualifications or acquiring a skill that was in demand was a way of circumventing low paid or insecure employment but that is far less certain now, and the advantages for graduates or skilled tradespersons are shrinking. So, in this context, it is understandable that young people are looking in the direction of virtual life as an arena in which to build a career. This may be true of body art enthusiasts, but similar tendencies can be seen amongst people aspiring to become professional online gamers, luxury goods reviewers, consumer electronics experts and much more.

Certainly, the dream of becoming a social media celebrity is not an easy or sure-fire way to earn a crust. For every high-level social media 'influencer' with a multi-million follower fan base, there are many more who have laboured long and hard in front of the webcam and got nowhere. The top earners are generally outliers, but this does not dampen ambition. Like winning a lottery, attaining a life-changing casino win or making it big in cryptocurrency, there is an enduring and pervasive appeal. Where body art is concerned, there are some interesting tensions in between the apparent 'bodies of subversion' sported by body art enthusiasts with digital capitalism and the dominance of social media companies in determining what can be seen, said or engaged with.

It is difficult to make sense of the opportunities and constraints presented by new digital cultures, or even to gauge whether we have the right kind of intellectual tools to comprehend the changes involved and how these changes shape and are shaped by our actions, desires, our work and our sense of who we are. This is not unusual in social and economic history. Often, new forms of production and consumption emerge before anyone really knows how they have become possible. Industrialisation, a move to factory production and progressive urbanisation had been developing in Europe and the United States for a long whilst before Marx called it 'capitalism'. People developed and were using money a long while before there was such a thing as a theory of money. Mechanically powered flight was achieved by people who were not exponents of an advanced theory of aerodynamics. This list of examples could easily be multiplied, but the point is that in some respects, intellectual life and science are downstream of material accomplishments.

So, is 'digital capitalism' the best metaphor for making sense of the profusion of digital life in the contemporary world? Yes, there are large companies involved and for those which have been lucky enough to supervene the profits are substantial. But there are some interesting conundrums too. Are we, the viewers and consumers the 'product', to be sold to advertisers, or are the online services which we consume the product, or is it the material that hundreds of millions of citizens upload to their social media account, or could it be something else entirely? Far from a nineteenth century model of bold entrepreneurs taking audacious business decisions which could lead to ruin or riches, governments tend to be the most significant economic actors in most richer nations. Economic life is propelled by a constant generation of central bank money, or 'quantitative easing'. At the same time, large companies and successful entrepreneurs can expound their own vision for our future civilisational direction via endowments, charitable donations, bodies such as the World Economic Forum and capture of policymakers and regulatory bodies. Even space programmes, once the preserve of superpower governments, are now the *mode du jour* for tech entrepreneurs and media magnates. Perspicacious readers may have spotted the similarity between what we have said here and the writings of economist and former Greek finance minister, Yanis Varoufakis. He promotes the term 'technofeudalism' to describe the symbiosis between tech companies, governments, the finance industry, content creators and consumers. In this view, the well-known large companies or online brands – Google, Facebook, Amazon, Apple, Twitter, TikTok and the like – are more similar to feudal lords than nineteenth century industrialists.

The relevance of this to the online world of body art concerns the way that so many practitioners and enthusiasts are making use of social media to promote their businesses, derive an income and form communities. In the techno-feudal world, these companies – or their armies of moderators and algorithm designers – have a good deal of power over what we can see, discover, talk about, upload or make a living from. In a sense, everything we see in online environments is there because the feudal lord or their functionaries want us to see it. On the other hand, material which they disapprove of is invisible, or at least much harder to find. Consequently, in an online environment, the body art entrepreneur must tread very carefully. You need to keep the public clicking, liking or following, and you need to attract an audience which is palatable to advertisers but, at the same time, material that is too risqué, off-message or which activates the designation of 'harmful' or 'disinformation' can incapacitate one's new business venture. In turn, the technofeudalists have a relationship with the national governments in the territories in which they operate, such that they are keen to appear like good technocratic citizens and not like troublemakers. Seeking to avoid further formal regulation, they may be particularly assiduous in hiding anything that might run counter to current policy priorities. Consequently, for anyone seeking to push the envelope of debate, possibility and practice the conventional web platforms may be a restrictive place. Avoiding 'cancellation', deplatforming or demonetisation or more insidious fates like 'shadow banning' can require some careful manoeuvring. Hence, the way that more contentious content is hidden away behind paywalls or new arrivals with a more explicit free speech ethos.

Consequently, the picture of body art we might gain from the online world is shaped by a number of forces extraneous to body art itself. It has enabled a great many exponents of the craft, who may be artists, canvases or both, to popularise the activity and even build careers in some cases. As well as Instagram stories or YouTube channels where content creators document their body art adventures, it shows up in other places too. The United Kingdom's parenting forum *Mumsnet*, not usually renowned for a cutting-edge approach to the human condition, has sub-forums concerned with body art – so the practice is finding its way into a whole variety of online media dealing with a number of different subject areas. This proliferation of material about body art across a variety of fora, facilities and platforms makes it hard to control, and this perhaps also reflects the ingenuity of people seeking to have conversations about this online in making themselves 'hard to kill'. If your YouTube videos are demonetised, you've still got your presence on a parenting forum, a Wiccan and Pagan forum and an Instagram, so you can build things up again. Oh, and maybe you can migrate the shorter items over to TikTiok and put the controversial stuff over on Rumble which has espoused a more explicit free speech ethos. These are just a few of the resources and platforms available today. No doubt there will be even more new ones along in the near future.

As well as navigating the algorithms and moderators of major social media platform, there would-be social media celebrity often depends for their livelihood on product placements and endorsements. Consequently, there is some interest in how marketers might decide which content creators they want to partner with and with whom they might want their items to appear. Whilst noting that modified or decorated individuals have struggled to gain credibility and trustworthiness in the past, Fernandes et al. (2022) claim that now there might be a 'tattoo premium' for product endorsing social media personalities. Those with body art can do better than those without, especially young women. Depending on the product and the target market, say Fernandes et al., it may be advantageous to consider associating products with more decorated social media influencers. This shows how marketing and monetisation have what Michel Foucault (1981) might have called a 'capillary' quality, that now body art is more acceptable and desirable; it is possible for it to be used to turn a profit. This, in turn, has the potential to shape the styles and expressions of body art found in the social media sphere, as people seeking to make a living at this sort of thing consider how they can best make themselves distinctive and agreeable to prospective advertisers.

Taking a different kind of online money-making as their focus, Kincaid et al. (2022) consider the role of body art in the viability of Kickstarter campaigns. Where there are visible tattoos in evidence in the campaigns' visual material, they did better and raised money more readily. The upshot of all this is that, in line with our theme of shifting boundaries in this chapter, body art is no longer marginal. In some commercial settings it can even be a positive asset. Business fashion has often been seen as rather small 'c' conservative field, with a lot of middle-aged men in grey suits. But in some cases, the more flamboyantly decorated individuals appear to have an advantage, as product endorsers or would-be entrepreneurs raising venture capital.

Moving off social media to conventional face-to-face activity, boundaries are shifting in a variety of human service fields too. Henle et al. (2021) described a study in which hypothetical applicants for hypothetical jobs were being judged based on their level of tattoo, from 'none at all' to 'highly visible'. The non-tattooed applicants were judged to be more employable and to merit a higher starting salary. However, findings like this are not reported everywhere, and there is also recent evidence that 'employees' visible tattoos may positively influence customers' attitudes and behavioural intentions toward products and some organizations through increased thoughts about the employee's artistic traits and competence' (Henle et al., 2021, p. 978). This may be especially true of an organisation seeking to cultivate an image of creativity and innovation. This emerging sense of advantage for decorated individuals, especially in creative fields, was also noted by Ruggs and Hebl (2022) in whose study, customers rated individuals with body art favourably. Hence, there is some emerging evidence that, as boundaries shift and body art emerges from the margins and takes over the centre ground, it is no longer a disadvantage in employment. A generation ago it was possible to hear people saying 'You'll never get a job' as a result of tattoos or piercings; now, *au contraire*, it might be an asset; a valuable piece of personal branding, especially in creative or innovative fields.

Where the presence of visible body art on people in human service roles is concerned, there has been a good deal of attention devoted recently to the effect of tattoos and piercings on patients' perception of health care personnel. With the growing popularity of body art across many different strata of society, it is no surprise that health care professionals have indulged too, either during their student days or later in life as they go through their careers. Consequently, there has been some interest in how their patients and their employers respond to this. Early work suggested some evidence to the effect that respondents generally have judged items like piercings and tattoos to be unprofessional or undesirable (Lill & Wilkinson, 2005; Menahem & Shvartzmann, 1998;

Westerfield et al., 2012). More recent material by Cohen et al. (2018), however, paints a more forgiving picture. Here, patients rated emergency room care by personnel with and without non-traditional piercings and tattoos or both. Patients' ratings did not indicate a difference in how they perceived physician competence, professionalism, caring, approachability, trustworthiness or reliability, whether or not they had exposed body art. Indeed, patients rated the attending physicians highly, no matter how they appeared. Interestingly, this study required some ingenuity to set up, as several of the participating physicians had to wear temporary tattoos and fake piercings some of the time as they were treating patients, and care had to be taken to cover up the tattoos of those who had genuine ones during the 'no body art' condition.

Writing in a personal opinion piece in the *British Medical Journal*, Bea Duric, a doctor with tattoos, describes how her own body art forms a point of connection and conversation piece with patients (Duric, 2022). Youngsters admire the bright colours, and even very elderly patients, whom one might expect to be a little more socially conservative, engaged in small talk about their grandchildren's body art. As Duric (2022) concludes:

> *personal style is what makes every doctor unique, a visual shorthand of our humanity and personhood. Whether it is through accepting and destigmatising tattoos, piercings, or neon hair, nurturing individuality makes happier doctors. (p. 1)*

A review of the situation in nursing by Pittman et al. (2022) reveals a similar picture, with concerns about the way that body art may be discouraged in organisational uniform and dress code policies, and lead to reduced perceptions of professionalism and competence on the part of patients and managers. On the other hand, as with Duric's observations above, there is a good deal of anecdotal evidence of body art being a talking point, a conversation starter and a means of building therapeutic relationships. Some nurses chafe against organisational rules which seem overly prohibitive, and good many patients do not appear to mind either way. So, perhaps the stage is set for some further emancipation amongst health professionals themselves.

Returning to the title of this chapter, concerned with shifting boundaries and movements from margin to centre, in the final part of this chapter let us consider a tension which often appears in experiences, accounts and academic literature about body art. That is, there is a tension between uniqueness and separation on the one hand and the desire for community and connection on the other. So, on one side we have people such as Rees (2021) writing about creating community and claiming authentic identity through body art. On the other hand, Weiller et al. (2021) talk about the need for uniqueness, especially in people with multiple conspicuous body modifications.

Perhaps on many people's body art adventurers there are elements of both uniqueness and distinctiveness and desire for communitas. This is illustrated in an early piece of work by Kathy Irwin (2001) showing the interplay between both these tendencies. In contrast to the stories of body art and body modification that emphasise difference, these kinds of decorations can just as readily be incorporated into the idea of the good citizen. Irwin (2001) showed how middle-class tattoo shop customers in a college town went to some lengths to legitimate what they were doing. For example, people described how their tattoos were carefully chosen, and how they had performed due diligence about the hygiene practices of the tattoo store. Participants also described their tattoos as a kind of rite of passage or a commemoration of a special event. In addition, the rationale people gave for their choice of design was carefully tied into their personal story, interests and commitments.

> Environmentalists chose images of mountain landscapes and trees, writers received images of characters in books, Greek mythology afficionados selected images of gods and goddesses, musicians got images of guitars and saxophones, and sports enthusiasts received images of their favourite teams or sports, such as bicycles, basketballs, or lacrosse sticks. (Irwin, 2001, p. 61)

Thus, tattoos often represented skills or capabilities valued in the wider society, and alignment with the values of education, the participants' parents and the wider world. It was as if, says Irwin, they were seeking to neutralise the possible stigma attached to tattoos.

This captures the very tension between margin and centre in body art. On the one hand people may want to signal their individuality, difference and personal style but at the same time there is a tendency to use body art as a way of signalling meanings and commitments that are much more widely shared amongst society as a whole too. Whilst some groups might frown upon tattoos, who could object to the cosy notion of strong family ties? Or the idea of people reading about classical mythology or playing sports?

This curious interplay between independence and integration, between individuality and communitarian values also plays out in the wider arena of fashion, style and consumption. With a large industry now surrounding body art, and its prominence in social media, as well as print and broadcast media and the cinema it is, in a sense a 'consumer item'. So how can we make sense of its role in these wider patterns of production and consumption?

Here too, when we consider the cultures of production and consumption the margin-centre tension is a conspicuous feature. To begin with, it is worth noting that recent consumer culture has a history of co-opting outsider styles, where fashions originating in youth subcultures become adopted by mainstream fashion brands and high street stores from the 1950s to the 1990s (Hebdige, 1979; Muggleton, 2000). This contrasts with an earlier but much longer period of history in which fashion worked in a top-down manner. The wealthy members of society drove fashion forward, and those who were less well-off created low budget versions or made do with cast offs and hand-me-downs. By contrast, in the twentieth and early twenty-first centuries, good many fashions originated from youth subcultures or perhaps from the working class as a whole. Jeans originated as miners' overalls and found their way to being a fashion item in hundreds of millions of wardrobes. Punk rock fashion items from the 1970s and 1980s found their way into *haute couture* via such luminaries as the late Vivienne Westwood. Latex and other high-shine fabrics have found their way out of the fetish club and into the celebrity wardrobe.

It could be argued that tattoos have undergone a similar transmutation. From something that was once the preserve of sailors, soldiers, motorcyclists and prisoners, they have become a desirable cool accessory for a much wider public. At the same time, in the last couple of decades, the role of youth subcultures as engines of sartorial aesthetic change has reduced somewhat, and instead the major corporate brands and fashion houses have seized the initiative. The mid twentieth century science fiction dystopias in which poor people sold advertising space on their bodies have come to be realised, but with the added twist that they themselves now pay for the privilege of advertising the company or design house on their clothes and accessories. As clothes have become the territory of large organisations, the body itself has become the canvas upon which the individual can work out some sort of aesthetic project.

Again, the margin-centre tension or dialectic is visible. As a number of writers on body art, such as De Mello (2000) and Atkinson (2002), have pointed out, there has been a middle-class appropriation of body art vectored through popular music and celebrities. As Atkinson (2002) puts it:

> In line with the sentiments of self-exploration, physical experimentation, and mind expansion ingrained in this era (1970s), dabbling in and with the socially avant-garde – including tattooing practices – became chic for the middle and upper classes. As countercultural icons, popular rock musicians, and cultural heroes were seen with tattoos, the young middle class started to frequent local tattoo parlors.
> (p. 44)

Although it was probably the 1990s and 2000s before this became more than a niche interest, the point is a telling one. The mainstreaming of body art represents something akin to a process of gentrification. The middle classes move in, but what happens to the people who already live there? Rich people enjoy dressing up as poor people, a bit like Marie-Antoinette. Accordingly, contemporary body politics has facilitated the redefinition of the tattoo as a legitimate and corporate-compatible medium of self-exploration, identity presentation and 'body work' for middle-class consumers (Strohecker, 2011).

Lest we create the impression that people with visible body art are just fatuous tourists or unthinking gentrifiers, displacing the working class and exoticising them as an 'other' like latter day imperialists, let us point out that these observations are in the manner of thought experiments. It's about asking where these ideas, techniques, practices and desires have come from and what it might mean for the people who originated them and those who adopt them. This doesn't mean that no one should have a tattoo unless they can demonstrate their working-class credentials. After all, how would we decide? What kinds of occupations and levels of deprivation would qualify? Moreover, there is an equally strong working-class tradition repudiating tattoos and viewing them as the marks of criminals and people with whom we wouldn't want to associate. Rather, this is an argument for taking a more reflective stance about what our body art means in the wider world. What interests does it serve? Who gets advantaged and who gets disadvantaged? Does it subvert or emancipate, or does it consolidate the broader impress of power? Does it separate or does it bring people together? It is this broader process of reflexivity or questioning which is valuable to foster, as well as willingness to hear other people's viewpoints, narratives and perspectives which might otherwise get overwritten by the dominant, corporate approved stories. It is this which will lead us to a full appreciation of the history and richness of the body art traditions and innovations which we appreciate, and recognitions of the human stories behind them.

7

THE HEALTH (AND BODIES) OF
BODY ARTISTS

In this chapter, we consider the health and wellbeing of artists, themselves. Whilst this is often not considered, this neglected topic has important implications for the viability and sustainability of body art in the future and its ability to provide career paths for those involved.

Let us first consider the health effects of working in the body art workplace. Like a good deal of repetitive physical labour, there are important implications for musculoskeletal health for body artists. There is potential for repetitive strain injury to backs, arms, wrists and eyesight. In addition, the long-term effects of vibration from equipment may be problematic. Whilst piercings are relatively rapid, tattoo artists may find themselves under pressure to schedule many long sessions in their working week, to earn a living or to meet demand from clients, with adverse consequences for their physical health.

In many nations, work design is subject to a variety of policy and legislation designed to improve health and safety – office workers, keyboard operatives and people using power tools in the construction industry have a variety of protections available to them. Yet, tattoo artists have very little access to this sort of support and often must work in ways which may be detrimental to their health. Indeed, federal regulations in the United States that specifically apply to the health and safety of body artists are sparse to non-existent. State-level regulations vary widely yet primarily pertain to licencing of artists and shops rather than workplace health and safety that prioritise artists' wellbeing. Similarly, in the United Kingdom, most regulations pertain to shops rather than ensuring the health and safety of artists themselves. When health and safety is prioritised, it often takes the form of sanitation and bloodborne pathogen protocol rather than ensuring access to quality health care and/or preventing injury/strain from repetitive motion. There is sparse literature on this topic (Grieshaber et al., 2012; Keester & Sommerich, 2017) with one study finding that tattoo artists are 'at an elevated risk for musculoskeletal problems', where their muscle activities far exceed recommended healthy limits (Keester & Sommerich, 2017, p. 142). However, organisations including the Coalition for Tattoo Safety (2022), actively advocate to standardise the industry and raise awareness of workplace health and safety issues for tattoo artists.

Insurance for *body art shops* is often mandated, whilst health insurance for *artists* often remains optional. Whilst healthcare in the United Kingdom is socialised, health insurance in the United States can be costly and often dependent on one's employment, with artists, who are often independent contractors rather than employees, electing to pursue insurance on the healthcare marketplace. 'Marketplace' health insurance coverage in the United States, obtained through the Department of Health and Human Services, is sometimes scant and variable in terms of services, providers, specialties and locations. Of course, the National Health Service (NHS) in the United Kingdom is not faultless despite guaranteeing cost-free/low-cost healthcare, with some individuals purchasing private insurance plans to obtain quicker and higher quality care. Thus, these often self-employed or contracted workers with physically demanding occupations and an enhanced likelihood of lifelong physical damage, and an arguably enhanced need for health services, are not guaranteed vital preventive nor acute healthcare access.

There are some practical and ergonomic improvements which may benefit members of the industry and yield better health and wellbeing for practitioners. Lack of ergonomic seating options and few breaks during the day is detrimental to artists' present and long-term health. Artists' schedules for breaks during tattooing vary in time and frequency, and this unpredictability of breaks is perhaps more pronounced for large-scale pieces requiring extensive time and attention to detail. Recently developed work chairs, including the NuChair (2023), prevent artists' spines bending and stop them from 'hunching' whilst tattooing by providing support for the front of the body rather than the back. Whilst these chairs promise relief from back pain and strain, they are not widely accessible and are quite costly at 650 USD each. Moreover, the way the chair is structured, with artists leaning the front of their torsos onto a structure akin to a seat-back (almost like a backwards office chair), does not accommodate artists with breasts very well. The chair is not easily transportable either, compromising the feasibility of tattooing in a convention setting or at another shop as a guest artist. This is not to say such ergonomic developments are unhelpful; rather, the case of this one chair reflects the broader, daunting challenge of addressing class-based and gendered disparities in body artists' health. For instance, travelling artists may not have the same steady stream of income as a shop-based artist, and travelling exacts wear-and-tear on the body. Much like overall healthcare, these artists likely have an arguably higher need for ergonomic chairs yet are less likely to be able to access them. Artists with breasts are often women artists who already face weathering (e.g. see Geronimus, 1992 for more about weathering) due to discrimination in the industry as detailed later in this chapter. Hence, maintaining physical health is even more crucial for marginalised artists who face health-related disadvantages in the field and in society, broadly.

As well as physical health, the emotional and cultural wellbeing of body artists is an issue of concern. The body art industry has often been somewhat sceptical of external scrutiny and has operated in a rather closed and cliquish manner. Part of this pattern can be attributed to the selectivity of the industry in accepting new artists. Historically, one's ability to tattoo and establish themselves as a tattoo artist has been determined through successfully seeking an experienced, expert artist who agrees to mentor an apprentice, and who has the time and resources to do so. The potential apprentice must convince said veteran artist of their skills in artistry whilst navigating the unspoken dynamics of likeability, showing utmost respect for the veteran's status and embodying an overall docile manner in exchange for learning from an industry expert (successful obtaining and deployment of cultural capital). The apprentice then closely works under that artists' guidance for an indefinite amount of time, the end of which is determined by the veteran artist. Moreover, some apprenticeships are paid, with the apprentice paying the master artist for their teaching, akin to paying tuition for university classes (Hunter, 2020).

Advances in technology have led to increasing access to resources that teach fundamentals of art and body art, and wider distribution of higher-quality work materials like inks and machines. Thus, there has been an increasing number of artists who are self-taught, eschewing exhausting, harrowing and long-term apprenticeships in favour of starting their own ventures. For these reasons and more, tattoo artists with fewer years of experience are often capable of producing high-quality body art that was unimaginable mere decades ago. With machines and inks more readily available than ever, thanks to Amazon and other online shopping outlets, along with video tutorials in generous supply, the landscape of body artists and training has changed greatly.

There have been stylistic shifts in the field of body art as well, changing from solely traditional work featuring bold lines and three colours of green, yellow and red, to neo/pop traditional artistry featuring the same bold lines and art style but with vivid hues. The field has also witnessed the growth of and advancement of hyperrealism, where tattoos look nearly identical to photographs. Bold lines have been joined by fine line tattooing featuring delicate, thin lines and precise detail. There has even been the advent of completely new styles including shimmering glitter tattoos and tattoos that look like patches one would wear on clothing. Nevertheless, body artists sometimes gatekeep and define what techniques and styles are more valid and authentic than others, repeating phrases like 'bold (lines) will hold' and quickly pointing out that hyperrealistic tattoos with few lines will surely fade or become unrecognisable over time (Arthouse Tattoo, 2021).

Indeed, artists with great skill yet fewer years of experience still face many challenges in the industry. Maintaining the 'master-apprentice' dynamic is thus still prevalent for both practical and cultural reasons. It maintains power structures, where this hierarchy is justified as 'paying dues' in the industry. Some artists have sought to make their teaching more accessible through efforts of teaching full courses online, including paid online 'universities' to learn tattoo techniques outside the realm of an apprenticeship. These efforts are often met with negative reactions ranging from mild annoyance to intense scrutiny and even mockery from some artists. Such criticism is not unwarranted, as such paid educational endeavours can also exploit customers and obscure the efforts and skill of industry experts (Midnight Moon Tattoo, 2020).

Self-taught artists remain marginalised in the body art community, and some of these concerns transcend cultural stigma. Historically, self-taught artists tended to be regarded as 'scratchers' who bought tattoo machines and would tattoo acquaintances at parties, or were incarcerated individuals using single needles and ink in non-sterile contexts, both being settings which increase the risk of infection and decrease the likelihood of a 'quality' art piece (Morrow, 2021). Whilst this still holds true, an increasing number of self-taught artists adhere to safety and hygiene protocol. Knowing the cultural cost of disclosing self-taught status as well, these artists tend to keep under the radar and may not disclose their self-teaching background for concern of being denied entry into the field (Morrow, 2021).

This has meant that those seeking to enter the field have historically been somewhat vulnerable, often having to undertake considerable periods of work unwaged in the form of apprenticeships. Apprentices are often 'the shop slave' (Molenaar, 2020), working gruelling hours and completing menial housekeeping tasks that are physically demanding. Artists describe a total absence of work-life balance, where they feel forced to neglect their families and other social relationships (Midnight Moon Tattoo, 2020).

Consequently, whilst in these apprenticeships, junior artists are vulnerable to exploitation, intimidation and sexual harassment. Often, entrants to the profession have been reluctant to report problematic behaviour from senior colleagues for fear of their future career prospects or possible retaliation (Farren, 2020). Such intimidation also alienates young artists from one another and may also turn them against each other. Amidst sexual harassment, assault and racism scandals amongst senior artists, new artists and apprentices have 'come out' about the abuse they experience in apprenticeships (Garland, 2020). However, there still remains pushback, as becoming more inclusive, accommodating and less abusive is sometimes seen as giving an 'unfair advantage' to new artists.

Allied to this is the question of how the community of practitioners responds to artists of colour who have often faced struggles for acceptance. Recent years have seen an increasing number of artists of colour in the field, yet these artists still face challenges resulting from implicit bias and explicit discrimination. Esteemed artists with the most experience tend to be white, cisgender men. This pattern, resulting from structural racism deeply embedded throughout society, then results in prioritising the tattooing of light skin tones. The techniques and colour palettes that are most effective on lighter skin tones are then considered objective, foundational knowledge in body art. Consequently, tattoo education centres on practice upon pale 'fake/practice' skin and white clients. Thus, there is a largely unshakeable belief – often framed as objective 'fact' – that 'dark skin is more difficult to tattoo', or 'bright pigments do not work/show up on dark skin' (Moyer, 2021). One artist encapsulates this school of thought in saying, 'Unfortunately, my style, technique, and ink sets I am using, they don't look good on darker skin tone' (see Moyer, 2021). Importantly, this artist is cognisant of other techniques and ink sets that may work better upon darker skin tones, but their training and experience clearly reflect the dominant paradigm that prioritises white skin. Well-known artist, Kat Von D, pushes further to justify her favouring white skin as a matter of scientific fact, elaborating

> *the truth is, depending on how much melanin concentration the client has, will depend on what pigments show up properly. It would be unethical to promise people with darker skin tones that pigments will heal properly and look the same as if they were tattooed on lighter skin tone, while taking their money' (quoted in Moyer, 2021)*

Von D, here, attributes the impossibility of utilising vivid pigments on dark skin to skin's melanin concentration, purporting to put the client's best interest first through specifying a desire to not 'take their money' for a fruitless attempt at providing a vivid tattoo. Importantly, this sentiment does not necessarily reflect any *conscious* bias – rather, this is what is presented as objective, neutral 'fact' in much of the industry (and, indeed, society overall).

Whilst framed as biological and value neutral, Von D's statement reflects the *social* phenomenon born of discrimination and marginalisation, rather than a simple phenotypical difference in skin tone (regardless of her individual intentions or conscious attitudes). The 'truth is' that tattooing originated in primarily indigenous cultures whose populations have darker skin tones. Indeed, artists of colour and their allies point out that it was when the tattoo industry became white-centric that darker skin become a 'problem' to tattoo. Tann Parker tells tattoo artists, 'You were taught that tattooing dark skinned people shouldn't be a thing, that people are too dark to get tattooed. You were taught that, and that's clearly wrong' (quoted in Moyer, 2021). Fortunately, there are good many artists who have not accepted this defeatist position and are working to improve the options available to customers with darker skin tones. Thus, there are – and always have been – techniques to tattoo dark skin in a way that allows vivid colours to appear bright and stand the test of time. Such techniques include simple attention to 'vibrancy shifts with different skin tones' (Moyer, 2021). Even changing the colour of a tattoo stencil from blue-based purple to red or green can make a tremendous difference (Moyer, 2021). Tattoo artists can also prioritise photography in natural light versus artificial light to allow these tattoos to look their best in photographs. So truly, many artists of colour note that it is a matter of re-incorporating and centring darker colours in fundamental colour theory during the tattoo education and training process. Because tattoo education and training are not standardised and because racism persists, there is no way to ensure such efforts will be regarded as valid, much less widely implemented.

Despite this widespread discrimination faced by both artists and clients of colour, body artists are making deliberate efforts to subvert the centring of white skin in the field. Often, these efforts are led by artists of marginalised statuses including artists of colour, queer artists and femme artists. For instance, artists will offer free 'colour tests' for clients with darker skin, so that the client (and artist) can see and be aware of how colours appear on their skin (Walker, 2021). Artists also post their techniques for tattooing darker skin online for free viewing and learning by fellow artists, including Jade Chanel's post on 'Tips on Tattooing Melanated Skin Tones' (Chanel, 2021) and Angel Rose's 'Dark Skin Tattoo Tips' (Morrow, 2021). Collectives such as the Shades Tattoo Initiative seek to 'build community and showcase the work of BIPOC tattoo artists' (Moyer, 2021; Snape, 2020). Ink the Diaspora features work by artists of colour on darker-skinned clients, spreading awareness regarding the barriers keeping artists of colour marginalised in the industry, and holding public panels with information on how artists can incorporate anti-racist practices into their work (Thorne, 2021).

Similarly, as more young women have sought to enter the field, they have often faced difficulties including lack of opportunity, not being taken seriously, and sexual harassment. Tattoo artist Gemma May (2022) poses the question on her Instagram account, 'How do we know that the Tattoo Artist sitting in that chair beside us is "safe"? We simply don't'. May is at the helm of the Tattooists Sexual Assault Survivor Support (TSASS) network, and movements such as #TattooMeToo have prompted women and femme body artists to speak out about mental, physical and sexual harassment and/or assault they have endured as apprentices and established artists (Garland, 2020). These artists will sometimes post about their experiences on their personal social media accounts (Hockaday, 2020), at times delving into great detail and naming their abusers. These artists recall experiences of groping from clients and fellow artists, having their tops involuntarily lifted whilst tattooing, being sexually assaulted and raped, being called names such as 'sluts' and 'whores' by their (often male) co-workers and more.

Courageously stepping forward, an increasing number of artists seek to help fledgling artists and the public alike distinguish between acceptable treatment or 'paying dues' and what is abuse in the body art industry. The overall culture of misogyny that pervades much of society prompts the public and industry alike to exercise intense scrutiny in response to these artists' brave and sincere vulnerability. Despite efforts like #BelieveWomen that urge people to first believe women's accounts of sexual harassment and abuse, rather than automatically doubting them, body artists recounting their experiences of abuse are often accused of lying about or embellishing their experiences (Farren, 2020; Garland, 2020; Hockaday, 2020). Consequently, artists sometimes disable commenting on corresponding social media posts or may 'fight back', sharing 'screen shots' of written communication with their abuser or others who acknowledged the abuse the artist endured.

Also in line with patriarchal structures, women and femme artists face increased pressure to maintain their physical appearance and beauty (Murray, 2017). For body artists, social media requires pristine pictures and videos of flawless tattoos. Consequently, for women and femme body artists, social media similarly requires themselves to appear faultless in beauty. Women and femme artists are scrutinised for their appearance, and others (particularly men), through illogical leaps and reaches, link women's appearance to their artistic skills. For instance, in a now-infamous exchange on the reality television show, *Ink Master,* a woman artist argued with a male artist about his skill in tattooing, to which he retorted, 'Why do you look 50 [years old] when you're 24 [years old]?' as if an insult to this artist's appearance would undermine her critique of his tattooing skills. Here, sexism intertwines with ageism, as both women and the elderly are viewed as incompetent and expendable.

Amid intense pressure to meticulously maintain appearances, in part to appease hegemonic expectations of feminine beauty, misogynistic double standards lead to accusations of women and femme artists unfairly wielding their 'erotic capital' (e.g., Hakim, 2010) to gain clientele and receive 'unwarranted' praise. In the body art industry (and society writ large), women's worth and reputation as artists rest on their physical appearance as much as it depends on their skill; both components must be faultless to compare to men of average skill regardless of their appearance.

Due to the same misogyny and cultural sexism that facilitates men having the right to control women/femmes and their bodies, social media users often direct message (DM) women and femme artists with graphic, sexual messages and unsolicited photos of their own naked bodies, often their genitalia. Women and femme artists sometimes cope with this harassment through dark humour.

For example, a woman tattoo artist founded an Instagram account, 'How Not to DM a Female Tattooer', beginning the account with screen shots from her own DMs accompanied by light-hearted or sarcastic captions that poked fun at the inappropriate messages. Soon thereafter, other femme body artists began submitting their own screen shots of lewd messages to the account where they would then join one another in the comment section to laugh at the ludicrous messages and the audacity of men who felt entitled to send them. These artists found empowerment in making public the messages of their abusers and pointing out how wrong and outright ridiculous these messages were. However, the humour and camaraderie quickly became too dark to sustain; the artist running the Instagram account shut it down somewhat suddenly, citing a harrowing experience of stalking that another tattoo artist experienced. Indeed, VKB followed this social media account, but due to its discontinuance, VKB was unable to find a citation to include here. The mental and emotional toll of this *one case* was enough to stop this *entire effort* in its tracks. Crucially, most tattoo artists know or have personally experienced a similar story to this stalking case. This case demonstrates the endless and pervasive harassment and abuse of women and femme artists on behalf of the industry and public alike. Facing such trauma at every turn makes resistance efforts difficult to maintain. Without a complete cultural overhaul of patriarchal structures, our best efforts to combat and overturn this mistreatment will remain incomplete.

A first step that artists and activists call for are regulations that ensure and allow law enforcement or other authorities to protect body artists and clients, along with mandatory background checks for all body artists (Lecklitner, 2021). Combined with the need for regulations to ensure ergonomic safety, body artists also tend to agree that there must be some degree of regulation and standardisation to ensure the health of all artists. As mentioned previously, artists have also started awareness of sexual harassment and assault through using the hashtag, #TattooMeToo. There now exist support networks, including the TSASS group and 'The Milieu Tattoo Union' that promotes inclusivity, equality and consent in the industry (Garland, 2020). Moreover, as is the case with many marginalised communities, there is a strong bond amongst 'lady tattooers', with an increasing number of shops being owned and occupied by women and femme artists who promise an environment of inclusivity, security and comfort. Similarly, the Instagram account, @ladytattooers, shares work by women and femme artists, providing a platform for their work to gain exposure and to expand their social networks with fellow artists.

With growing twenty-first century awareness of queer, trans and nonbinary issues, questions arise as to how these communities fare in a field which has hitherto often been quite hegemonically masculine and heterosexual. Whilst the arts and crafts of body art practice have sometimes offered career opportunities for young nonconformists of every gender, the process of forging an identity and making a living is not always straightforward. Indeed, despite an increasing number of queer-owned shops, transphobia and homophobia abound in the industry, ranging from 'casual' discrimination in the form of microaggressions to more explicit discrimination and violence. There is an overall pattern of queer artists being less likely to obtain apprenticeships, which means more queer artists are self-taught, compared to their straight and/ or cisgender counterparts. This leads to a higher prevalence of stick-and-poke style tattoos amongst queer artists, a polarising style subject to scrutiny in the industry.

Queer-owned shops are often occupied by solely or predominantly queer artists with a devoted attention to queer and otherwise marginalised clientele (Momeni, 2022; Schade, 2022). Queerness, by nature, is intersectional and transcends discrete categorisations. Hence, queer-owned shops often centre the needs of disabled populations, populations of colour and fellow queer clients (Momeni, 2022; Schade, 2022). Indeed, Samantha Sasso (2021) observes that 'slowly but surely, a movement of artists – specifically artists who identify as queer – are subverting the subculture to create a community that welcomes all marginalized bodies'. The queer shop setting often mimics the 'chosen family' dynamic of queer communities in society, broadly; if outcasted by biological family, queer communities form 'chosen families' of close, trusted relations who may not be biologically related but whose love and support are unconditional (Sasso, 2021).

The seemingly simple action of posting an 'all bodies welcome' sign on a shop door or banner on a shop's website, for instance, signals to all clients that their bodies and very identities will remain unquestioned, understood and indeed embraced in their current state. Queer artists tend to understand, with sympathy or empathy, the hatred and discrimination that queer, Black, brown, disabled and/or scarred bodies face in society. Some queer shop owners thus completely overhaul the traditional shop setup that features several tables in an open space, electing to, instead, include privacy dividers throughout the shop between tables or even have individual, private tattooing rooms. Shop owners might also follow a booking schedule that allows for only one client in the shop at a time, so as to centre client privacy, confidentiality and comfort.

These shops, then, become places of sensitivity, sanctuary and healing. For instance, getting a chest tattoo is a wholly different experience for a transgender person who has had 'top surgery' (removal of breast tissue), compared to a client whose gender aligns with their sex assigned at birth. These tattoos are part of a path to liberation; the overall understanding of reclaiming and celebrating one's body through body art holds an even deeper meaning for bodies that have been societally deemed 'wrong' by their nature. Understanding the gravity and significance of this process, some queer artists and shops employ trauma-informed techniques, which may include providing squeeze balls for clients, opportunity to take multiple breaks and even a sensitive space for clients to cry. For marginalised clientele, tattoos are genuinely therapeutic, and queer artists prioritise making their shops, schedules and approaches part of that therapy process.

Another effort to centre marginalised communities includes keeping tattoo costs low or cost-free for clients of colour as a form of reparations. Whilst there may be an arguably enhanced need for queer artists to be paid fairly for their labour in light of the discrimination they face, these same artists also recognise that granting access to the body art community via low-cost or cost-free tattoos might be the only way for marginalised populations to obtain this healing and therapeutic form of bodily adornment.

In the preceding chapter, we considered the challenges facing people seeking to develop and maintain a presence in the new digital environments afforded by social media platforms. Artists too are at the mercy of the algorithm, and may feel a compulsion to be perpetually present in these arenas promoting and maintaining their profile, which can place them under a great deal of pressure. The rise of social media has afforded newfound freedom for artists yet is simultaneously constraining and controlling. Smartphones have made it easier to take and post high-quality photos, sharing them widely to local and international audiences. Because artists can take multiple photos and select the best ones therefrom, keeping portfolios updated is arguably less arduous than it has been historically. Sharing photos of tattoos on social media facilitates widespread attention and following, allowing for a stream of customers and facilitating connections amongst artists.

Findings from recent research (Force, 2022) are echoed in artists' accounts of their experiences on social media. The process of self-branding, building devoted clientele and posting images to social media requires intensive efforts. The question of how a particular piece of work will play on social media and how it will fare in terms of the social media company's algorithms can be as important as how it will look in the flesh. Artists spend tremendous time and energy taking photos and deciding which one looks best before posting it, accounting for angles and lighting, all whilst enduring the mental gymnastics of considering how it will fare on social media. Indeed, the unspoken laws of social media are ever evolving, with a recent shift in public favour from still images to short videos in the form of TikToks or Instagram reels that take intensive technical and cultural knowledge to create. Artists must be keenly aware of factors such as what time of day to post, which days of the week to post, and how often to post to garner the most attention and positive feedback. Further, discourse in the form of memes and perishable pop culture is constantly changing: a sound bite from a funny video may make for impactful audio in a video one week whilst using it in subsequent weeks (or even days) may be met with annoyance, exasperation or 'cringe' from audiences. Fascinatingly, artists often include brief clips of their faces in these videos, as the algorithm is more likely to promote videos that include human faces. Indeed, there is more to worry about now than 'convention lighting' or glare when selecting images to share with the world.

Indeed, browsing is fleeting; artists must secure that 'double-tap' or 'like' of approval from users who otherwise quickly scroll past their painstakingly constructed social media post. Artists' success *outside* of social media is increasingly determined by success *within* social media. Body artists' duties and expectations differ from social media 'influencers' whose income is what they post and create on social media – their entire career is in that virtual space. Nathan Molenaar (2020) elaborates,

> *As a new artist, I considered my hours to be 24/7. I needed to build up my clientele, and that meant spending a ton of time on social media, talking to potential customers. If they messaged me at 2 am, and I didn't respond ... someone else might. Now that I have a steady stream of clients, though, I don't have to be quite as on top of that.*

Body artists must therefore engage intently on social media and then continue their tireless efforts 'in real life', efforts further requiring artistic creativity and technical precision. Further blurring the divide between digital leisure and 'real life' work, artists have largely transferred administrative components like booking and inquires to online spheres as well, significantly increasing their online workload (Force, 2022).

Thus, whilst social media has disrupted historical hierarchies that were once solely reliant upon years of experience, along with training under and recognition by esteemed veterans, it has also created immense burden: (1) leaving talented artists who are unable to access or deftly understand social media relatively unrecognised and (2) exponentially burdening and exhausting younger, emerging artists whose habitus is oriented towards social media. Consequently, social media has not undone *the* need for social capital so integral to industry success; rather, the parties from which artists draw their social capital have shifted from solely industry experts to social media users as well.

8

TOWARDS ACHIEVING THE BENEFITS OF BODY ART

In this chapter, we will begin the concluding section of the book by considering how the benefits of body art may be fully realised and the possible impediments to this being achieved. We have considered earlier how body art may be used to mark the life-course, how it might be used to indicate recovery and reclamation, may contribute to social relationships and ways of making a living as well as representing a sort of body capital. We have hinted at how it might contribute to therapeutic relationships of a more conventional kind. Whilst getting a tattoo or piercing may never make it into the official guidance from medical organisations, we hope to have shown how body art contributes to the quality of lives of those who indulge in this activity and perhaps even the people around them.

One of the major impediments to achieving the full potential of body art as a way for enhancing health, wellbeing and resilience comes from the health professional and research communities themselves. We have hinted at this earlier in the book, but it is worth spending a little time familiarising ourselves with the full force of this disapproval, because even in the third decade of the twenty-first century, it is apt to colour the experience of modified or decorated individuals seeking health care, and affect the way they are represented in academic writing as well as popular media and policy debates.

There has been a long history of health professionals exhibiting somewhat sceptical or even hostile attitudes to body art. Perhaps this is related to a sense that they are called upon to put right infections or allergic reactions incurred by failed attempts at body art. As we shall see, some body art enthusiasts report experiencing negative reactions from health professionals, even when seeking healthcare for other kinds of problems unrelated to their body modification. Indeed, sometimes this was felt to be more censorious than the healthcare response to people who'd sustained injuries playing sport or other hazardous recreational activities. However, recent years have seen some shifts in professional concerns and sensibilities, and the experience now is generally much more positive, with health professionals often sporting body art of their own.

As an example of the kind of research which positions body art fans as irresponsible and risk-prone, let us consider a large UK-based study in 2005 which canvassed over 10,000 participants, of whom just over 100 had a piercing other than an earlobe (Bone et al., 2008). Young women aged between 16 and 24 were particularly strongly represented in this group, with just over 46% reporting such a piercing. Popular sites included the navel (33%), the nose (19%) and parts of the ear other than the lobe (13%). Rather less prevalent were the tongue and the nipple (both 9%) and eyebrow, lip and genitals were 8%, 4% and 2%, respectively. Amongst young men, the prevalence was a little different, with tongue and nose piercings being less popular.

This study by Bone et al. (2008) is also worthy of mention because it is often the origin of high estimates of piercing complications which are regularly repeated in the wider literature and in popular advice, suggesting that nearly a third of piercings result in complications. Study of the article itself, however, reveals that complications were quite generously defined and included swelling and bleeding which are not unusual with any minor wound. Even for the 0.9% stating that they attended hospital as a result, as this is self-report, it is not clear whether they required high-intensity treatment only obtainable in hospital, or whether the adverse effects could be managed more prosaically, with some reassurance and topical antibiotics. In the United Kingdom, it is sometimes easier to obtain medical care by turning up at a hospital Accident and Emergency (A&E) department than obtaining a general practitioner (GP) appointment. This is not officially encouraged, so as to leave Emergency departments free for more severe injuries, but it is a common practice amongst the population, thus visits to A&E are not necessarily an indicator of severity. Whilst the after-effects of piercings may be concerning and non-trivial, it is important to look at how the figures were compiled.

Even so, reading the descriptions of piercing in the medical and nursing literature, one might easily think that severe injuries were involved. Here is a passage from Hoover et al. (2017) concerning piercings where cartilage is involved. These, they say,

are at a much higher risk of wound complications than those done through soft tissue. The perichondrium is stripped from the cartilage at the wound edges, and microfractures of the cartilage occur during piercing. These injuries lead to oedema and bleeding into the cartilage. This causes decreased blood circulation to relatively avascular tissue and increased susceptibility to infection. (Hoover et al., 2017, p. 525)

This passage is then followed by dire warnings about piercings becoming infected. Now, we are not encouraging readers to take risks with their health, but there seems to be almost a zest for the worst-case scenario. In everyday life, the mundane experience is much more likely to be that piercing in the upper part of the ear, for example, are a bit less comfortable to lie on in bed, are a little more likely to secrete fluid and take longer to fully heal than those in fleshier areas. Whilst the injuries and sites are a little different, the burden on the human frame and its immune system is comparable to that of myriad everyday minor injuries such as grazed knees from falling over, skinned knuckles and scratches from gardening, strains or sprains and impact injuries from playing sport. It is possible for severe consequences to ensue, but generally they don't.

In the practice of heath care, there are many meticulously well-behaved patients, a number of whom suffer a good deal of pain and disability, of which a proportion, sadly, is iatrogenic. Healthcare itself may be a source of infection (Brown et al., 2008, 2014). So, there is something interesting going on here whereby it is the changes brought about by the person's own volition that are the problem. It is as if the health care professionals and researchers feel like they have a monopoly over the human body and what can and cannot be done with it. This reminds one of us (BB) of an incident in the early 1990s when he mentioned to a young woman that he had pierced his nipples. She was aghast; 'You're not supposed to do that. I'm a biologist. You're not supposed to do that,' she shrieked. Fortunately, BB found this merely amusing at the time, but what is interesting is that she construed her biology degree as lending her authority over what people were supposed to do, or rather not do, with their bodies. This also perhaps illuminates the observations we have made above about how the putative hazards of cosmetic body piercings are construed. This goes beyond the physical risks and extends into a proprietorial attitude towards what is allowable with the body. Indeed, these examples echo Michel Foucault's (1973) concept of the medical gaze, where all that is needed in order to identify bodily pathology is the practitioner's (or, in this case, any scientist's) sight and examination of the body; patient input is irrelevant and unimportant in defining what is pathological and what is normal or desirable. This then invites a range of interesting philosophical issues about who really owns the body. In some cases, it doesn't seem to be the person inside it!

In thinking about realising the potential of body art, a further issue emerges when we consider how body art researchers have conceptualised and investigated the issue. There are some curious points of inflection in the literature which point to the intriguing and sometimes deeply gendered way in which writers and researchers think about their participants. For example, one of our observations when reading around the subject for writing this book was how both the field itself and the academic scholarship around it has conceptualised gender. There are some rather odd omissions here, and the area is therefore ripe of some new thinking as well as novel practical and research direction. The first is that where people have written about body artists themselves, they overwhelmingly tend to be writing about men. Women's experience as artists and practitioners in this growing industry is often a side note – yes, they have a hard time, and that's about all we hear. There are some notable exceptions, such as Margot Mifflin's *Bodies of Subversion* (Mifflin, 2013), although this is more focussed on women as recipients or wearers of tattoos than as artists. This omission is all the more striking given the prominence that some women have achieved in the field as practitioners, celebrities and authors, with names like Kat Von D and Madame Chinchilla making inroads into the popular consciousness, and Elayne Angel's (2021) *Piercing Bible* growing ever larger through its multiple editions. Even though body art has attracted the attention of feminist scholars, from the broadly supportive (e.g. Dann, 2021; Pitts, 2003) to the highly critical (Jeffreys, 2000), it is still difficult to find detailed ethnographic accounts of women making inroads into the field as artists or business owners (for an exception, see Yuen Thompson, 2015). Women, it seems, are seen as the canvas rather than the artist.

In the light of this, for any would-be postgraduate student or academic seeking to do ground-breaking work in the area, a study of women artists would make a fantastic original project. Thinking about the social sciences more broadly, there is still much to be done to adequately grasp and study women's agency, ingenuity and determination. So, in some ways it is no surprise that this lacuna has appeared in relation to body art as well. It took us a little while to spot this too – sometimes when an item is missing entirely, it is difficult to notice that it is not there!

Following this theme of the curiosities of gender in relation to body art, one area where women do show up a good deal in the literature is concerned with their experience as recipients (Dann, 2021). The material we have covered earlier in this book about reclamation, self-definition and empowerment as well as recovery after illness has included the experience of women extensively. Whilst in some cases researchers have included mixed samples, there is nevertheless a great deal of focus on women and meaning-making in relation to body art. This prompted us to wonder about the meaning and purpose of body art amongst men, and whether anyone had studied this. However, if we look for literature about young men and body art, material is much sparser. Moreover, it tends to look at men from 'outside', rather than from the point of view of lived experience, and positions them as a problem. For example, there are references to gang-affiliated tattoos in young men (Kubik, 2019) and the desirability of getting them removed (Kimmel, 2020; Ojeda et al., 2023), or in conjunction with their membership of far-right organisations (Miller-Idriss, 2017). This tendency to look at men from the 'outside' is sustained across other lines of scholarship too. There is a thriving strand of research where participants are asked to judge male figures with and without tattoos. Typical findings include the perception that tattooed men are seen as more aggressive, dominant and masculine (Galbarczyk et al., 2020).

You could therefore read the literature and come away with the impression that women are hard at work making meaning, healing or reclaiming, and men are in prison. Or at least they are apt to be hyperaggressive, far-right affiliated individuals who will probably end up there sooner or later. We are painting in broad brush strokes here, but the caricature is not far off the mark. It reflects the old childhood folk rhyme of girls being made up of 'sugar and spice and all things nice' versus boys being a combination of 'slugs and snails and puppy dogs' tails'. Perhaps this has emerged because many women inspired by feminist scholarship have found occupational homes in the academy and have been understandably keen to investigate women's experience, including in relation to body art, especially as women tend to be treated as objects of study rather than subjects with agency, motivations and desires. For the research community looking at men, matters have remained much like the olden days, with tattoos showing up in forensic contexts, just like in the time of Cesare Lombroso (1896). Lombroso, it might be remembered, was a renowned nineteenth century Italian criminologist who viewed criminals as atavistic links or throwbacks to our earlier 'savage' evolutionary history; they were thus more likely to communicate pictorially than through language. Whilst his strongly social Darwinist conception of crime is no longer so popular, the agendas he set have still not entirely disappeared.

This relative quietism about men's experience of body art is all the more curious, because clearly in other topic areas men's experiences are investigated. It is not too hard to find accounts of men trying to make progress in boxing, bodybuilding and in their careers, or even as fellow sufferers when their partners have miscarriages. Rather than adduce long lists of references for these topics we invite the reader to have a look for themselves. So, it is not as if male experience is entirely opaque. Rather, it does not appear that anyone is looking at it in this field. Once again, this might make a productive thesis topic or research programme for anyone seeking to make a name for themselves in the area.

Whilst on the subject of the curiosities surrounding gender and body art, it is also noticeable that illness, or at least recovery from it, is celebrated in the literature on women and embodiment. The breast cancer recovery tattoos which have been studied in detail and which we have mentioned earlier in this book are good examples. Yet once again, with men, this does not appear to be a large-scale phenomenon, or at least not one which has been studied. There is, as far as we know, no great enthusiasm for tattoos to commemorate, say, penile or prostate cancers. Even though breast cancers may sometimes occur in men, there is yet to develop a tradition of body art memorialising them or the sufferer's recovery. Indeed, cancers of the penis and prostate still hold the stigma that breast cancer once had, for example in Audre Lorde's (1980) day where breast cancer was still a heavily stigmatised topic that weakened 'morale', before breast cancer awareness efforts became ubiquitous, simultaneously infantilising (e.g. fluffy pink ribbons and teddy bears) and sexualising breasts (e.g. 'save the tatas' and 'save second base') in a way that is more publicly palatable than the reality of being ravaged by cancer. Whilst there are efforts around prostate and penile cancer awareness, these are much less pervasive and men's embodied experiences of cancer are few and far between (Chapple & Ziebland, 2002), let alone how they make meaning and find liberation through body art or modifications.

These curiosities seem to have emerged from the way that people think about men and women or male and female sex roles in wider society and this has then informed the way researchers go about looking at body art, and perhaps also how body art wearers or consumers think of themselves as decorated individuals. These gender-related examples show how, rather like a searchlight, our tacit theories of what people are like, what happens and what matters helps to give shape and form to experience and the kinds of research findings which are generated. Therefore, a more reflective approach concerning the gaps and omissions in our knowledge may well benefit the quest to realise the full range of benefits from body art.

Returning for a moment to the impediments to achieving the full potential of body art as a medium in the health humanities, let us now explore a little further the way in which academics and health-care personnel have often taken a dim view of body art. Indeed, this sense of body art as somehow subversive or transgressive has perhaps added to its appeal in some quarters. Whilst this chapter is attempting to focus on the achievable benefits of body art, it is worth detailing this body-art-sceptical tradition in a little more detail. As we have noted with the earlier mentions of body art related injuries, it's easy to find material emphasising the pathology and risk of body art. It is important to grasp this because overcoming it is key to fully achieving the benefits of body art. It is also worth being forewarned about all this especially if you are a decorated person, because it may well emerge in interactions with doctors, nurses, therapists and teachers. The more exuberant expressions of body art – and sometimes even the more discreet ones – may occasion disapproval, and it is valuable to understand how this has happened and where it comes from. In the face of disapproval, it is useful to remember that the disapprover is not inevitably correct, no matter how august their professional credentials or how they cloak their disapprobation in therapeutic expertise.

The field of psychoanalysis has a long history of undermining and discounting the ideas, desires and personal narratives of those who are not initiates of its arcane mythos. Not surprisingly, its adherents have also provided a rich source of material for scholars seeking to represent body art in derogatory terms. An early example of this comes from Grumet (1983) who theorised that people obtain tattoos in order to compensate for low self-esteem. He argued that tattoos represented 'a psychic crutch aimed to repair a crippled self-image, inspire hope, keep noxious emotions at bay, and reduce the discrepancy between the individual and his aspirations' (Grumet, 1983, p. 491). In similar vein, Karacaoglan (2012) described what she saw to be the unconscious motivations for tattoos, and claimed that 'the painful penetration of the skin in the process of tattooing ... is a form of acting out' (p. 24) and proposed that tattoos symbolise 'an attempt to actively represent and recompense, as it were, an early deficiency' and a 'dialectical record of the mother-father relationship' (p. 25). She described the process of tattooing for the recipient as masochistic, adding that tattooing was an alternative form of expression that patients 'resort' to when unable to verbalise 'unendurable affect' through language. Karacaoglan (2012, p. 27) concluded that tattooing was a 'form of perversion'. Any resemblance to Cesare Lombroso's thinking over a century earlier is probably not co-incidental!

It is worth looking closely at how writers in this school of thought formulate the issue. It is as if there is a very narrowly defined range of 'proper' feelings and appropriate kinds of action, and anything outside this expert-approved realm is some kind of wrongdoing. Moreover, there is an underlying premise that the expert knows the patient (everyone is a 'patient' in traditional psychoanalysis!) better than they can possibly know themselves. The patient's inner workings are laid bare before the astute clinical gaze (e.g. Foucault, 1973). This is revealing not because any of it is necessarily true, but because it shows how a group of so-called caring professionals can abrogate to themselves a kind of moral and epistemological privilege that is immune to countervailing experiences or narratives. Of course, people with body art can be unhappy, distressed or disoriented, just like anyone else, but what is interesting here is how their decorations are seen as a kind of symptom, rather than as, for example, identity, connection or strength.

The situation does not have to be like this, of course. It is possible to use psychoanalytic theory in more benign ways to tell the story of the life trajectory and add interpretive richness to the practices of body decoration. Indeed, the high symbolism of many tattoo designs lends itself to some of the more baroque interpretations which may be possible. This more playful approach, recognising the metaphorical quality of much interpretation – and a good deal of psychoanalysis itself – can be fun and mutually enhancing.

In the late twentieth century, there was a good deal of other work going on which similarly sought to interpret body art as a kind of pathology, though without some of the more florid interpretive language found in psychoanalysis. A paper by Harry (1987) said that tattoos were a risk factor for self-harm in a population of male offenders. Based on a sample of 21 people with tattoos and 24 without, he noted self-harm scars on the tattooed inmates. From this he deduced that '…tattoos, despite their ostensibly decorative quality, may be a form of self-mutilation' (Harry, 1987, p. 171).

A further example in similar vein comes from Farrow et al. (1991), where amongst clients of a drug treatment programme it was found that people with tattoos had 'low self-esteem, delinquency, drug abuse, family and peer modelling, and participation in satanic rituals' (Farrow et al., 1991, p. 184). They then go on to say that tattoos should be addressed as a health problem by medical professionals. This tendency has continued into the more recent past. For example, Carson (2014) associated tattoos with early mortality, explaining this as being because people with tattoos were disproportionately likely to die from drug overdoses or meet with violent deaths. Koch et al. (2016) found a higher level of self-reported suicide attempts in young adults with multiple tattoos, especially young women. In addition, those with multiple tattoos experienced higher self-esteem, too. Koch et al. (2016) describe this finding as 'paradoxical', but it could indicate that the process of acquiring and wearing body art has some kind of therapeutic value to the owner. This possibility is not pursued, however.

There is a good deal more literature like this. It would take quite a whilst to list it all, but the handful of examples above should give an indication of the overall tenor of the material that has dominated the discourse, and which has built the careers of 'experts'. Keagy (2017) provides a useful table of material she had found up to 2016, and no doubt more could be adduced from the last few years. This kind of work, with similar assumptions and conclusions was widely performed in the late twentieth and early twenty-first centuries, often with similar limitations. It was often concerned with highly specialised (as well as marginalised and disempowered) individuals, often in institutional contexts and frequently based on small samples. Nevertheless, authors readily supposed that the observations made of vulnerable people in institutional contexts were true of the wider population. In the majority of such work, the academic interest in body art focussed specifically on people who had come to the attention of the authorities because of some sort of problem. They were in drug treatment programmes, institutions for troubled young people or young people in trouble, such as forensic facilities and psychiatric clinics.

As Keagy (2017) points out, most of this work starts from a priori assumptions that body art is a problem, or at least a diagnostic sign of something more sinister. Some kinds of body modifications, perhaps especially tattoos, are more likely to be found amongst people from the working classes or who are otherwise on low incomes. In most nations, this is associated with poorer health outcomes and lower life expectancy. In the United States – but to some extent in other countries too – it may be difficult for those on low incomes to access health care. If body modifications really were responsible for lowering life expectancy, worsening morbidity and condemning the wearer to long periods in prison or psychiatric hospital, this would make them extraordinarily powerful, worse than smoking, drinking or drug use. However, before we jump to any hasty conclusions about body art having adverse consequences, it is important to note some limitations of this kind of work. As many of these studies are correlational, there may be a whole host of unexplored variables that yield the observed associations. The experience of adverse life events, trauma and unexplored differences in circumstances may all make a difference to health outcomes. We have already mentioned social class, but there could be a great many more. Until more subtle multivariate research in this field comes into vogue, we simply will not know. However, there are some suggestions emerging in the literature that as body art becomes more widely enjoyed amongst young adults that the observed correlations are lessening. So, the relationships that were seen in the 1980s may be harder to pinpoint four decades later.

Another constraint on interpreting research which claims that body art derives from some sort of traumatic event or unhappy childhood comes from personal experience of how people generally talk about adverse experiences. Not everyone will disclose that they have been sexually abused or raped in response to a self-completed survey. Only a very small minority of those who have survived this kind of experience will tick the box or fill in a free text response about it on a questionnaire. This is the sort of thing that is more likely to come up in conversation with a good friend or within a well-established therapeutic relationship rather than in a questionnaire survey. So, the possibility exists that what we are seeing is a difference in self-disclosure. Maybe people with body art are more attuned to their bodies and what has happened to them and are more willing to disclose about adverse events, including in their responses to a questionnaire study. This is speculation on our part, but it is worth bearing in mind when reading about the purportedly greater rate of adverse experiences in the owners of body art. These data are almost invariably derived from self-reports.

Despite all these limits on interpretation, there is some evidence that these negative attitudes persist on the part of some health professionals, who may well assume the worst when presented with people who have body modifications. This appears even when people are attempting to consult health professionals about problems unrelated to their body art. Keagy (2017) interviewed body-modified participants who had attempted to seek treatment for other health problems and found their difficulties interpreted through the lens of their body art. One young woman who was suffering from a complaint that was eventually diagnosed as mononucleosis described her journey through the healthcare system as follows:

> Q: *Are you implying that they thought that you had an STD because of [how you looked]?*
>
> A: *I think so. Because I got tested for HIV and AIDS more times than any 19-year-old I know …. So I had a total of 17 doctor visits and 11 blood panels done [panels of tests for STDs] over a couple of months and was tested for HIV and AIDS. This was all from a bunch of different doctors, because nobody was ever telling me anything or doing anything for me, more than telling me to take ibuprofen which – they were telling me my liver enzymes were triple what they should be. And they were saying it was because I was drinking. I was not drinking. I hadn't touched alcohol in months because I was so sick, I couldn't even move. I was like, 'I'm not drinking'. Anyway, so basically different doctors making me take pregnancy tests and STD tests. […] I had to medically withdraw from my classes that semester. I had to quit one of my jobs. The last doctor, one female doctor out of, I want to say it was probably like seven or eight doctors total, was the only one who didn't make me take a pregnancy test, didn't make me do an STD panel, and just immediately was like yeah,*

> *that's absolutely what you have. Because every time I'd*
> *be like 'I think it's mono' and they'd be like, 'Well, let's*
> *do a test and let's do this...' I got tested for vitamin D*
> *deficiency on top of it, too. Like, really? You think I'm*
> *not getting enough vitamin D. (Keagy, 2017, p. 599)*

This sounds very like a phenomenon called 'diagnostic over-shadowing', which has been noted in studies of mental health patients. Complaints which would elicit further investigation and assessment in people without a psychiatric history are often interpreted as part of the mental health problem in people with a mental health problem. It is as if the presence of body art elicits a range of stereotypes which may be misleading – that the person has a drug problem, engages in high HIV risk activities and the like, and that's what the health problem 'really' is.

In addition to unhelpful stereotyping, Keagy's (2017) participants described not being offered local anaesthesia for wound suturing, feeling like they're being treated like a 'junkie', who was seeking hospital grade pain killers, or being used as an example to take pictures of. It could sometimes take a long time to access care, even once they had arrived at hospital. One participant described how he

> *was in an emergency room and this guy just refused to*
> *treat me for hours, like eight hours. They just left me*
> *laying in the emergency room. And I felt like I was dying.*
> *And the reason why is because it was my second time in*
> *there for it and I don't go to any medical unless I have to –*
> *I hate it – and I literally couldn't see. Photosensitivity, all*
> *kinds of shit. I couldn't even use my phone. And this guy –*
> *it's my own assumption, but I think it had something to*
> *do with that [how he looked]. (Keagy, 2017, p. 600)*

Indeed, some people had more or less given up on seeking conventional health care and favoured complementary and alternative approaches as they found them to be a more accepting environment. In many clinical facilities, attendees have to spend a good deal of time waiting around irrespective of whether they are bearing body art or otherwise, and they may feel that their treatment had been perfunctory and unsuited to their concerns. Even the 'best-behaved' patients, who would not dream of allowing a needle to penetrate their skin unless it were in the hand of a health professional, suffer from long waits and a good deal of pain and impairment, too. So, in some ways these are 'equal opportunity problems'. However, amongst many of the people whose experiences are reported here there is a lingering suspicion that some of the delays and the rather off-beam diagnostic avenues pursued owed a good deal to their prominent body art.

This chapter is entitled 'Towards Achieving the Benefits of Body Art' yet we realise a good deal of what has been covered comprises material about things that may militate against this. Negative views expressed in the academic and clinical literature, adverse experiences in health care and a miasma of risk and dire consequences have been cultivated in a variety of disciplines. However, it is worth reviewing these experiences here because they are instructive and show how the attitudes of those in positions of trust and expertise may prevent the full benefits of body art to be realised. The negative attitudes of days gone by might be softening, especially as health professionals themselves may have body art collections, or at least may have had some exposure to these activities during their student days. Thus, perhaps the seeds of change have been sown.

The other reason why we have detailed this material is because it reveals something interesting and perhaps profound about the way knowledge, science and medicine work and their relationship to the wider society of which they form a part.

The social formations termed 'science' are often not about facilitating human potential and freedom but rather attempting to place constraints on it. The bulk of professional effort and expertise where body art is concerned is devoted not to solving the problems but to diminishing the decorated person and issuing portentous warnings. Relatively little official effort has been devoted to extending the repertoire of activity that can be enjoyed safely. We more or less take this for grated these days. We are warned to keep our body mass index between certain expert-approved limits, to give up smoking, take more exercise, reduce our carbon footprint, eat less sugar, not allow our dogs to foul the footpath and not to leave it 'too late' to have children, amongst many other things.

This is not true in all fields of science or medicine. For example, in HIV medicine, many practitioners have actively embraced the mission to enable hedonism, enjoyment and intimate life to take place whilst reducing risk (Brown & Jaspal, 2022). Treatment and preventative measures have been developed to enable infection risk to be reduced and viral load to be diminished so as to facilitate a more manageable approach to sexual life. The dire warnings and the sense of an HIV diagnosis as a death sentence are now things of the past in many nations.

There is something here that is missing from the vast majority of medico-scientific writing on body art. In HIV medicine, it is much easier to find an attitude of being in the service of the patient group and their aspirations for a low-risk love life. Rather than giving us peasants a good telling off, the HIV physicians and researchers in Brown and Jaspal's (2022) study described how they were working to make a better life possible for their patients without any diminution of pleasure and spontaneity. This orientation struck Brown as very refreshing and was reminiscent of an earlier age where science and medicine were conceived of as facilitating human aspirations rather than revising expectations downwards. Where HIV is concerned, some problems remain to be solved, for example, the question of whether 'undetectable equals untransmittable' applies to a parent wishing to breast- or chest-feed, but even so, there is a distinct sense of therapeutic optimism in this field.

Knowledge and expertise don't merely reflect the world around us but are often profoundly normative and moralistic. They are frequently deployed in the sense of telling people to do certain things and not others. In a sense, a good deal of the medico-scientific literature is stuck in this phase. Thinking ahead to a more utopian future, it would surely not be hard for researchers and clinicians to adopt the same sort of orientation towards body art as HIV specialists do towards their patient group. There is all manner of opportunities for genuinely creative and facilitative collaborations where body art is concerned.

In this vein, the example we gave earlier in the chapter about body artists, of tattooists working to offer a better range of opportunities and colour palettes to clients with darker skin tones, is redolent of a similar spirit of ingenuity and optimism. We do not have to take the supposed 'facts' of a situation for granted. These can instead be seen as challenges to be transcended.

To consider a couple of further examples, in much the same way as the immune system is most effective not in sterile conditions but if it is regularly stimulated to act against pathogens and allergens, perhaps the decorated body learns new ways to address the intrusions and modifications which can enhance our understanding of healing and natural reconstruction. Rather than being a nuisance, the tendency of the body to migrate piercings towards the surface and remove them has much to tell us about how it 'decides' what it wants to eject and what it wants to keep. The experience gained in such collaborative inquiry could be useful from the point of view of research on transplants and implants. These are just speculations, but they highlight the possibility of conjoint working on problems of mutual interest. It is perhaps through mutual exploration of these moments of 'wild surmise' that the full benefits of body art might be realised.

9

CONCLUSION: THE MULTIPLE ARTS OF THE BODY REVISITED

We hope the preceding chapters have given the reader a sense of some of the kinds of body art available and some of the ideas, debates, meanings and practices around it. As this is deliberately intended to be a short volume, we have provided at best a sketch of what is happening. Both the academic literature on which we have drawn and the field of practice are changing month by month, so this is merely a snapshot. By the time you, the reader, reach this text a good deal of it is likely to be out of date. We have even made some suggestions about changes we would like to see in the future ourselves. However, there are some more enduring themes and ideas which we hope will provide thinking tools for anyone interested in the field of body art, how it intersects with the health humanities and the possible benefits it might bring.

A well-explored theme in the literature and by those who have recovered from illnesses is the use of body art to symbolise their illness and their survival of it. This is particularly well developed in the literature on breast cancer, but it could equally well be applied to other illnesses. This will probably never be recommended as an official form of therapy and will not feature in health professionals' codes of conduct, but we can be reasonably confident that this confers some benefit, at least judging by the stories of those with lived experience. It may therefore be valuable for practitioners to explore with clients possible artistic solutions and ameliorations to life changing illnesses or injuries. Body art can enable a sense of recovery or reclamation. Perhaps this might be easier to cope with and less risky and invasive than some kinds of conventional reconstructive surgery. Anecdotal evidence and personal experience suggest that, for the right person, it might be as effective as psychotherapy to help in coming to terms with losses or impairments. Something that builds on patients' or clients' interests, beliefs or which enjoys some meaning personal symbolism is most likely to be of value.

This theme of meaning underlies a great many other accounts of body art – there are stories of people commemorating events in their life course such as birthdays, graduations, starting a family and much more. There are many tales of tattoos that represent important things in a person's life – commitments, passions and pastimes. This tendency to ascribe meaning is very widespread, and it would be easy to gain the impression that body art comes about as a result of deeply meaningful and intentional decision making. It doesn't have to be like this of course. BB chose his body art because he liked the look of it, and people asking about the meaning seem nonplussed when he doesn't have a story about it. However, the stories told about the meaning of body art are a near-ubiquitous feature.

One facet of the changing face of storytelling about body art is its proliferation across a variety of digital spaces including stand-alone websites and social media platforms. People seeking to make a living in these new media must play a complex game with the proprietors and moderators of social media platforms. This may involve attempting to avoid getting demonetised or deplatformed on one hand, and also trying to reverse engineer the algorithms so as to enable their profile to be presented to a wider range of consumers. This sophisticated digital choreography is a game which people seeking to succeed under what has been called 'digital capitalism' or 'techno-feudalism' must become good at. Whilst the people we have mentioned who are currently making places for themselves in the social media sphere at the time of writing may come and go, the longer-term task of making sense of these new environments and the livelihoods they afford will remain with us for some time to come. The multiple arts of the body include that which is inscribed on the skin, but also what is presented across social media platforms.

Body art is developing a higher profile in everyday life and, even appearing amongst health and social care professionals, there is an increasing number of individuals sporting body art. This may not, as was originally feared, result in patients or clients having a lower opinion of them and their capabilities. An Instagram post from endometriosis surgeon, Andrea Vidali, featured a picture of himself with his tattooed arms on full display, sarcastically captioning the photo: 'Never ever consult a doctor with tattoos'.

This contrasts with a long history of body art being thought of by researchers and health professionals as indicating something wrong with the bearer. Criminal tendencies, drug problems, unresolved trauma and mental ill health have all been inferred, sometimes all at the same time. Whilst the more overtly stigmatising attitudes and inferences from research are less conspicuous nowadays, this still remains a stumbling block. As we have noted, this contrasts with the therapeutic optimism visible in some other areas of medicine, and with the ingenuity and dedication with which body artists are expanding the scope and inclusiveness of what is possible.

Body art can enable connections and social relationships across generations – older adults' interest in tattoos has brought them into contact with the younger generation who are practising body art. This tackles loneliness and isolation and promotes intergenerational learning. Sometimes this might also activate mutual cross generational interests – motorcycling or music being obvious ones – and areas of commonality. As we have argued earlier, it is unique in its potential to build relationships, perhaps especially amongst people who might not see themselves as candidates for conventional psychotherapy or counselling. For people who find social interaction difficult, or who are anxious in asking for what they want, the sense of direction offered by gaining a much-desired piece of body art has been a powerful motivator in overcoming these sources of hesitation. People acquiring body art can be thought of as adding to their bodily capital and body art enthusiasts and practitioners are exploring new territory both in the exploration of what is possible and in contributing to personal and collective wellbeing. It may fairly be said that body art offers a way of creating happiness and social solidarity beyond what can be achieved through medicine and the therapeutic disciplines alone.

REFERENCES

Aguayo-Romero, R., Reisen, C. A., Zea, M. C., Bianchi, F. T., & Poppen, P. J. (2015). Gender affirmation and body modification among transgender persons in Bogota, Columbia. *International Journal of Transgenderism, 16*, 103–115.

Allen, D. (2017). Moving the needle on recovery from breast cancer: The healing role of postmastectomy tattoos. *Journal of the American Medical Association, 317*(7), 672–674. doi:10.1001/jama.2017.0474

Allen, A. (2016). *The end of progress: Decolonizing the normative foundations of critical theory*. Columbia University Press.

Angel, E. (2009). *The piercing Bible: The definitive guide to safe body piercing*. Crossing Press.

Angel, E., & Saunders, J. (2021). *The piercing Bible: The definitive guide to safe body piercing*. Crossing Press.

Antoninetti, M., & Garrett, M. (2012). Body capital and the geography of aging. *Area, 44*(3), 364–70.

Arthouse Tattoo. (2021). *Tattoo style: The trouble with realism*. https://arthousetattooaustin.com/tattoo-style-the-trouble-with-realism/

Atkinson, M. (2003). *Tattooed: The sociogenesis of body art*. University of Toronto Press.

Atkinson, M. (2002). Pretty in ink: Conformity, resistance, and negotiation in women's tattooing. *Sex Roles, 47*, 219–235.

Atkins, R. (1991). *Artspeak*. Abbeville Press Inc.

Atkinson, M., & Young, K. (2001). Flesh journeys: Neo primitives and the contemporary rediscovery of radical body modification. *Deviant Behavior, 22,* 117–146.

Barker, R. G. (1968). *Ecological psychology: Concepts and methods for studying the environment of human behavior.* Stanford University Press.

Bergland, A., Fougner, M., Lund, A. & Debesay, J. (2018). Ageing and exercise: building body capital in old age. *European Review of Aging and Physical Activity, 15*(7). https://doi.org/10.1186/s11556-018-0195-9.

Bly, S., Gwozdz, W., & Reisch, L. A. (2015). Exit from the high street: An exploratory study of sustainable fashion consumption pioneers. *International Journal of Consumer Studies, 39*(2), 125–135. https://doi.org/10.1111/ijcs.12159

Bone, A., Ncube, F., Nichols, T., & Noah, N. D. (2008). Body piercing in England: A survey of piercing at sites other than earlobe. *British Medical Journal, 336*(7658), 1426–1428. https://doi.org/10.1136/bmj.39580.497176.25

Bordo, S. (1993). *Unbearable weight.* University of California Press.

Botz-Bornstein, T. (2012). Female Tattoos and Graffiti. In R. Arp (Ed.), *Tattoos philosophy for everyone: I ink, therefore I am* (pp. 53–64). John Wiley & Sons.

Bourdieu, P. (1978). Sport and social class. *Social Science Information, 17*(6), 819–840.

Bourdieu, P. (1984). *Distinction: A social critique of the judgement of taste* (R. Nice, Trans.). Harvard University Press.

Bourdieu, P. (1986). The forms of capital. In J. G. Richardson (Ed.), *Handbook of theory and research for the sociology of education* (pp. 241–258). Greenwood Press.

Bourdieu, P. (1997). Bodily knowledge. In P. Bourdieu (Ed.), *Pascalian meditations* (pp. 129–163). Stanford University Press.

Breuner, C. C., & Levine, D. A. (2018). Adolescent and young adult tattooing, piercing, and scarification. *Pediatrics, 141*(2), e201773630.

Brown, B., & Baker, S. (2012). *Responsible citizens: Individuals, health and policy under neoliberalism.* Anthem Press.

Brown, B., Crawford, P., Nerlich, B., & Koteyko, N. (2008). The habitus of hygiene: Discourses of infection control in nursing work. *Social Science and Medicine, 67*(7), 1047–1055.

Brown, B., & Jaspal, R. (2022). Imaginaries of patienthood: Constructions of HIV patients by HIV specialist health professionals. *Sociology of Health and Illness, 42*(6), 972–990. https://doi. org/10.1111/1467-9566.13472

Brown, B., Tanner, J., & Padley, W. (2014). 'This wound has spoiled everything': Emotional capital and the experience of surgical site infections. *Sociology of Health and Illness, 36*(8), 1171–1187. https://doi. org/10.1111/1467-9566.12160

Caliendo, C., Armstrong, M. L., & Roberts, A. E. (2005). Self-reported characteristics of women and men with intimate body piercings. *Journal of Advanced Nursing, 49*(5), 474–484. https://doi. org/10.1111/j.1365-2648.2004.03320.x

Carson, H. J. (2014). The medium, not the message: How tattoos correlate with early mortality. *American Journal of Clinical Pathology, 142*(1), 99–103.

Chanel, J. (2021). *Tips on tattooing melanated skin tones.* https://www. instagram.com/p/CKEzTfrBnup/

Chapple, A., & Ziebland, S. (2002). Prostate cancer: Embodied experience and perceptions of masculinity. *Sociology of Health & Illness, 24*(6), 820–841.

Coalition for Tattoo Safety. (2022). *Coalition for Tattoo Safety: Who we are.* https://coalitionfortattoosafety.org/about/

Cohen, M., Jeanmonod, D., Stankewicz, H., Habeeb, K., Berrios, M. & Jeanmonod, R. (2018). An observational study of patients' attitudes to tattoos and piercings on their physicians: The ART study. *Emergency Medical Journal, 35*, 538–543. doi:10.1136/emermed-2017-206887.

Crossley, N. (2001). *The social body: Habit, identity and desire.* Sage.

Dann, C. (2021). *Navigating tattooed women's bodies: Intersections of class and gender.* Emerald Publishing Limited.

Dann, C., & Callaghan, J. (2019). Meaning-making in women's tattooed bodies. *Social and Personality Psychology Compass, 13,* e12438. https://doi.org/10.1111/spc3.12438

Dann, C., Callaghan, J., & Fellin, J. (2016). Tattooed female bodies: Considerations from the literature. *Psychology of Women Section Review, 18,* 43–51.

DeMello, M. (2000). *Bodies of inscription: A cultural history of the modern tattoo community.* Duke University Press.

De Mello, M. (2007). *Encyclopedia of body adornment.* Greenwood Publishing Group.

Dickson, L., Dukes, R. L., Smith, H., & Strapko N. (2015). To ink or not to ink: The meaning of tattoos among college students. *College Student Journal, 49*(1), 106–120.

Duric, B. (2022). Erasing the stigma: Tattoos in the medical workforce. *British Medical Journal, 378,* o1744, http://dx.doi.org/10.1136/bmj.o1744.

Durkheim, E. (1915). *The elementary forms of the religious life.* The Free Press.

Eubanks, V. (1996). Zones of dither: Writing the postmodern body. *Body & Society, 2*(3), 73–88.

Fabius, C. (1998). *Mehndi: The art of henna body painting.* Three Rivers.

Farren, M. (2020). *Inside the toxic tattoo industry: Symbols to sexual assault.* Dazed Beauty. https://www.dazeddigital.com/beauty/article/51184/1/tattoo-metoo-industry-reform-nazi-symbols-racism-sexual-assault-accountability

Farrow, J. A., Schwartz, R. H., & Vanderleeuw, J. (1991). Tattooing behavior in adolescence. A comparison study. *American Journal of Diseases of Children, 145*(2), 184–187.

Fernandes, T., Nettleship, H., & Pinto, L. H. (2022). Judging a book by its cover? The role of unconventional appearance on social media influencers effectiveness, *Journal of Retailing and Consumer Services*, 66. https://doi. org/10.1016/j.jretconser.2022.102917

Force, W. R. (2022). Tattooing in the age of Instagram. *Deviant Behavior*, 43(4), 415–431.

Foucault, M. (1981). *Power/knowledge: Selected interviews and other writings*. Harvester.

Foucault, M. (1973). *The birth of the clinic: An archeology of medical Perception*. Vintage Books.

Garber, M. (2015). How badass became a feminist rally cry. *The Atlantic*. https://www.theatlantic.com/entertainment/archive/2015/11/how-badass-became-feminist/417096/

Giles-Gorniak, A. N., Vandehey, M. A., & Stiles, B. L. (2016). Understanding differences in mental health history and behavioral choices in a community sample of individuals with and without body modifications. *Deviant Behavior*, 37(8), 852–860.

Galbarczyk, A., Mijas, M., Marcinkowska, U., Koziara, K., Apanasewicz, A., & Ziomkiewicz, A. (2020). Association between sexual orientations of individuals and perceptions of tattooed men. *Psychology and Sexuality*, 11(3), 150–160.

Garland, E. (2020). The tattoo industry is facing 'a reckoning.' *Vice*. https://www.vice.com/en/article/bv87gd/tattoo-industry-sexism-racism-uk

Geronimus, A. T. (1992). The weathering hypothesis and the health of African-American women and infants: Evidence and speculations. *Ethnicity & Disease*, 2, 207–221.

Giddens, A. (1991). *Modernity and self-identity: Self and society in the late modern age*. Stanford University Press.

Gilligan, C. (1977). In a different voice: Women's conceptions of self and of morality. *Harvard Educational Review*, 47(4), 481–517. https://doi. org/10.17763/haer.47.4.g6167429416hg5l0

Goffman, E. (1963). *Stigma: Notes on the management of spoiled identity*. Houghton Mifflin.

Goldberg, S. (2018). For Decades, Our Coverage Was Racist. To Rise Above Our Past, We Must Acknowledge It. *National Geographic*, March

12. https://www.nationalgeographic.com/magazine/article/from-the-editor-race-racism-history

Grieshaber, D. C., Marshall, M. M., & Fuller, T. (2012). Symptoms of Musculoskeletal Disorders among Tattoo Artists. In *Proceedings of the Human Factors and Ergonomics Society 56th Annual Meeting.*

Grumet, G. W. (1983). Psychodynamic implications of tattoos. *American Journal of Orthopsychiatry, 53,* 482–492.

Hakim, C. (2010). Erotic capital. *European Sociological Review, 26*(5), 499–518.

Hardy, D. E. (1988). *Tattoo time: New tribalism.* Hardy Marks.

Harris, J. (2017). Centering women of color in the discourse on sexual violence on college campuses. In J. Harris & C. Linder (Eds.), *Intersections of identity and sexual violence on campus: Centering minorized students' experiences* (pp. 83–100). Stylus Publishing Inc.

Harry, B. (1987). Tattoos, body experience, and body image boundary among violent male offenders. *Bulletin of the American Academy of Psychiatry Law, 15*(2), 171–178.

Hebdige, D. (1979). *Subculture: The meaning of style.* Routledge.

Heelas, P. (1996). Introduction: Detraditionalization and its rivals. In P. Heelas, S. Lash, & P. Morris (Eds.), *Detraditionalization: Critical reflections on authority and identity* (pp. 1–20). Blackwell.

Henle, C. A., Shore, T. H., Murphy, K. R., & Marshall, A. D. (2021). Visible tattoos as a source of employment discrimination among female applicants for a supervisory position. *Journal of Business Psychology, 37,* 107–125. https://doi.org/10.1007/s10869-021-09731-w

Hesse, R. W. (2007). *Jewelry making through history: An encyclopedia. Handicrafts through world history.* Greenwood Publishing Group.

Hobsbawm, E., & Ranger, T. (1983). *The invention of tradition.* Cambridge University Press.

Hockaday, J. (2020). Tattooists 'quit jobs in shame' over 'inappropriate' messages to female clients. *Metro.* https://metro.co.uk/2020/06/06/

tattooists-quit-jobs-shame-inappropriate-messages-female-clients-12813513/

Hoover, C. V., Rademayer, C.-A., & Farley, C. L. (2017). Body piercing: Motivations and implications for health. *Journal of Midwifery and Women's Health*, 62(5), 521–530. https://doi.org/10.1111/jmwh.12630

Howson, A. (2004). *The body in society.* Polity Press.

Hunter, D. (2020). *Are tattoo apprenticeships paid?* Authority Tattoo. https://authoritytattoo.com/are-tattoo-apprenticeships-paid/

Hutson, D. J. (2013) 'Your body is your business card': Bodily capital and health authority in the fitness industry. *Social Science & Medicine, 90*, 63–71.

Irwin, K. (2001). Legitimating the first tattoo: Moral passage through informal interaction. *Symbolic Interaction, 24*(1), 49–73.

Jeffreys, S. (2000). 'Body Art' and social status: Cutting, tattooing and piercing from a feminist perspective. *Feminism and Psychology, 10*(4), 409–429.

Joseph, J. (1992). *Selected poems.* Bloodaxe Books.

Lecklitner, I. (2021. The Movement to Reclaim Ink from Abusive Tattoo Artists. *MEL Magazine.* https://melmagazine.com/en-us/story/tattoometoo-recovery-artists-tattoo-abuse

Lorde, A. (1980). *The cancer journals.* Penguin Random House.

Karacaoglan, U. (2012). Tattoo and taboo: On the meaning of tattoos in the analytic process. *International Journal of Psychoanalysis, 93*, 5–28. https://doi.org/10.1111/j.1745-8315.2011.00497.x

Karupiah, P. (2013). Modification of the body: A comparative analysis of views of youths in Penang, Malaysia and Seoul, South Korea. *Journal of Youth Studies, 16*, 1–16.

Katz, J. (1988). *Seductions of crime: Moral and sensual attractions in doing evil.* Basic Books.

Keagy, C. D. (2015). *Healing marks: Body modification in coping with trauma, identity, and its ramifications for stigma and social capital* [Ph.D. dissertation]. Department of Sociology, University of California, San Francisco.

Keagy, C. D. (2017). Institutional constructions of medical stigma and its perception by multiply body-modified individuals seeking treatment. *Deviant Behavior, 38*(5), 593–604. https://doi.org/10.1080/01639625. 2016.1197582

Keester, D. L., & Sommerich, C. M. (2017). Investigation of musculoskeletal discomfort, work postures, and muscle activation among pracitcing tattoo artists. *Applied Ergonomics, 58*, 137–143.

Kimmel, M. (2020). *Healing from hate: How young men get into-and out of-violent extremism.* University of California Press.

Kincaid, P. A., Short, J. C. & Wolfe, M. T. (2022). Got ink, get paid? Exploring the impact of tattoo visibility on crowdfunding performance. *Journal of Business Venturing Insights, 17*, https://doi.org/10.1016/j. jbvi.2022.e00317

Klein, R. (2016). Chosen scars: Breast cancer and mastectomy tattooing as digital feminist body politics. In B. Ashton, A. Bonsall, & J. Hay (Eds.), *Talking bodies. Vol II* (pp. 191–220). Palgrave Macmillan.

Klesse, C. (2000). '"Modern primitivism": Non-mainstream body modification and racialized representation', In M. Featherstone (Ed.), *Body modification* (pp. 15–38). Sage.

Klesse, C. (1999). 'Modern primitivism': Non-mainstream body modification and racialized representation. *Body & Society, 5*, 15–38.

Kluger, N. (2012). Piercings génitaux: épidémiologie, aspects socioculturels, sexualité et complications. *Presse Medicale, 41*, 21–31.

Koch, J. R., Roberts, A. E., Armstrong, M. L., & Owen, D. C. (2016). Tattoos, gender, and well-being among American college students. *The Social Science Journal, 52*(4), 536–521. https://doi.org/10.1016/j. soscij.2015.08.001

Kosut, M. (2006). An ironic fad: The commodification and consumption of tattoos. *Journal of Popular Culture, 39*(6), 1035–1048. https://doi. org/10.1111/j.1540-5931.2006.00333.x

Kubik, J. (2019). *The impact of gang involvement, tattoo presence and a new diversion program on juvenile recidivism outcomes* [Ph.D. thesis]. Rutgers University.

Kukkonen, I. (2021). Physical appearance as a form of capital: Key problems and tensions. In O. Sarpila, I. Kukkonen, T. Pajunen, & E. Åberg (Eds.), *Appearance as capital* (pp. 23–37). Emerald Publishing Limited. https://doi.org/10.1108/978-1-80043-708-120210002

Lane, D. C. (2017). Understanding body modification: A process-based framework. *Sociology Compass, 11*, e12495. https://doi.org/10.1111/soc4.12495

Leader, K. (2016). "On the book of my body": Women, power, and "tattoo culture". *Feminist Formations, 28*(3), 174–195. https://doi.org/10.1353/ff.2016.0048

Lecklinter, I. (2021). The tattoo industry has a predator problem – And a controversial solution. *Mel Magazine.* https://melmagazine.com/en-us/story/pre-employment-background-checks-tattoo-industry

Lill, M. M., & Wilkinson, T. J. (2005). Judging a book by its cover: Descriptive survey of patients' preferences for doctors' appearance and mode of address. *British Medical Journal, 331*, 1524–1527.

Lodder, M. (2011). The myths of modern primitivism. *European Journal of American Culture, 30*(2), 99–111.

Lombroso, C. (1896). The savage origin of tattooing. *Popular Science, 48*, 793–803.

Lamont, E., Roach, T., & Kahn, S. (2018). Navigating campus hookup culture: LGBTQ students and college hookups. *Sociological Forum, 33*, 1000–1022.

Madfis, E., & Arford, T. (2013). The dilemmas of embodied symbolic representation: Regret in contemporary American tattoo narratives. *Social Science Journal, 50*(4), 547–556. https://doi.org/10.1016/j.soscij.2013.07.012

Maira, S. (2000). Henna and hip hop: The politics of cultural production and the work of cultural studies. *Journal of Asian American Studies, 3*(3), 329–369.

Martin, C. R., & Cairns, S. L. (2015). Why would you get that done?! Stigma experiences of women with piercings and tattoos attending postsecondary schools. *Canadian Journal of Counseling and Psychotherapy*, *49*, 139–162.

May, G. [@gemmaymayy]. (2022, March 18). *How do we know that the tattoo artist sitting in that chair beside us is 'safe'? We simply don't* [Photograph]. Instagram. https://www.instagram.com/p/CbPS1blMIHf/?utm_source=ig_web_copy_link

McLuhan, M. (1951). *The mechanical bride: Folklore of industrial man.* Vanguard Press.

McNay, L. (1999). Gender, habitus and the field: Pierre Bourdieu and the limits of reflexivity. *Theory, Culture & Society*, *16*(1), 95–117.

Mears, A. (2015). Girls as elite distinction: The appropriation of bodily capital. *Poetics*, *53*, 22–37.

Menahem, S., & Shvartzman, P. (1998). Is our appearance important to our patients? *Family Practice*, *15*, 391–7.

Metzger, D. (1997). Tree. In *Tree: Essays and pieces*. North Atlantic Books.

Metzger, D. (1988). I am no longer afraid. In L. H. Lifshitz (Ed.), *In her soul beneath the bone: Women's poetry on breast cancer* (p. 71). University of Illinois Press.

Midnight Moon Tattoo. (2020). *Sorry, we have no apprentices today.* https://midnightmoontattoo.com/sorry-we-have-no-apprenticeships-today/

Mifflin, M. (2013). *Bodies of subversion: A secret history of women and tattoo* (3rd ed.). Simon and Schuster.

Miller-Idriss, C. (2017). Soldier, sailor, rebel, rule-breaker: Masculinity and the body in the German far right. *Gender and Education*, *29*(2), 119–215.

Miserandino, C. (2003). *The spoon theory*. https://butyoudontlooksick.com/articles/written-by-christine/the-spoon-theory/

Molenaar, N. (2020). *I worked at a tattoo shop for 10 years and can tell you exactly what it's like*. Tattooing 101. https://tattooing101.com/learn/tips-advice/working-in-a-tattoo-shop/

Momeni, T. (2022). LGBTQ+ tattoo studios provide safe spaces for marginalized groups. *The Baltimore Banner*. https://www.

thebaltimorebanner.com/culture/lgbtq-tattoo-studios-provide-safe-spaces-for-marginalized-groups-EDDW57HUZ5DTVJDZAQBULEBQNI/0

Morello, S. J., Gustavo, M. S., Moreno, D., Engelmann, S., & Evangel, A. (2021). Women, tattoos, and religion an exploration into women's inner life. *Religions, 12,* 517. https://doi.org/10.3390/rel12070517

Morrow, J. (2018). *Knowledge is power, or is it? An essay on self-taught tattoo artists.* Tattoo Do. https://www.tattoodo.com/articles/knowledge-is-power-or-is-it-an-essay-on-selftaught-tattoo-artists-14015

Morrow, J. (2021). *Dark skin tattoo tips.* Tattoo Do. https://www.tattoodo.com/articles/dark-skin-tattoo-tips-150199

Moss, A. (2021). Your favourite tattoos on Instagram are probably faked. *Vice.* https://i-d.vice.com/en/article/88gab3/instagram-tattoos-fake

Moyer, A. (2021). Black & white but white all over:Colourism in the tattoo industry. *Spring: A Magazine of Socialist Ideas in Action.* https://springmag.ca/black-white-but-white-all-over-colourism-in-the-tattoo-industry

Muggleton, D. (2000). *Inside subculture: The postmodern meaning of style.* Berg.

Murray, G. (2017). *This is what it's really like being a woman in the tattoo industry.* Refinery 29. https://www.refinery29.com/en-us/2017/05/156273/woman-tattoo-artists-sang-bleu

Myers, J. (1992). Nonmainstream body modification: Genital piercing, branding, burning, and cutting. *Journal of Contemporary Ethnography, 21*(3), 267–306.

Naudé, L., Jordaan, J., & Bergh, L. (2017). 'My body is my journal, and my tattoos are my story': South African psychology students' reflections on tattoo practices. *Current Psychology, 38,* 177–186.

Neveu, E. (2018). Bourdieu's capital(s). In T. Medvetz & J. Sallaz (Eds.), *The Oxford handbook of Pierre Bourdieu* (pp. 347–374). Oxford University Press.

NuChair. (2023). *Why NuChair?* Retrieved February 26, 2023, from https://nuchair.com/pages/why-nuchair

Ojeda, V. D., Magana, C., Hiller-Venegas, S., Romero, L. S., & Ortiz, A. (2023). Motivations for seeking laser tattoo removal and perceived outcomes as reported by justice involved adults. *International Journal of Offender Therapy and Comparative Criminology*, 67(1), 126–145.

Orbach, S. (1978). *Fat is a feminist issue*. Paddington Press.

Oultram, S. (2009). All hail the new flesh: Some thoughts on scarification, children and adults. *Journal of Medical Ethics*, 35(10), 607–610.

Pittman, A., Gary, J., & Pepper, C. (2022). An integrative review of body art in nursing. *Nurse Educator*, 47(4), 197–201. https://doi.org/10.1097/NNE.0000000000001168

Pitts, V. (2003). *In the flesh: The cultural politics of body modification*. Palgrave Macmillan.

Portwood-Stacer, L. (2012). Anti-consumption as tactical resistance: Anarchists, subculture, and activist strategy. *Journal of Consumer Culture*, 12(1), 87–105. https://doi.org/10.1177/1469540512442029

Rees, M. (2021). *Tattooing in contemporary society: Identity and authenticity*. Taylor and Francis.

Reich, K. (2018). *Surplus Values: A New Theory of Forms of Capital in the Twenty-First Century*. University of Cologne Press.

Reid De Jong, V. (2022). Unveiling beauty: Insight into being tattooed postmastectomy. *Nursing Forum*, 57, 536–544. https://doi.org/10.1111/nuf.12714

Roggenkamp, H., Nicholls, A., & Pierre, J. M. (2017) Tattoos as a window to the psyche: How talking about skin art can inform psychiatric practice. *World Journal of Psychiatry*, 7(3), 148–158.

Rosenblatt, D. (1997). The antisocial skin: Structure, resistance, and "modern primitive" adornment in the United States. *Cultural Anthropology*, 12(3), 287–334.

Rubin, A. (1988). *Marks of civilization: Artistic transformations of the human body*. University of California Press.

Rudschies, C. (2022). Power in the modern 'surveillance society': From theory to methodology. *Information Policy*, 27, 275–289.

Ruggs, E. N., & Hebl, M. R. (2022). Do employees' tattoos leave a mark on customers' reactions to products and organizations? *Journal of Organizational Behaviour, 43*. doi: 10.1002/job.2616

Said, E. (1978). *Orientalism*. Pantheon.

Samadelli, M., Melis, M., Miccoli, M., Vigl, E. E., & Zink, A. R. (2015). Complete mapping of the tattoos of the 5300-year-old Tyrolean Iceman. *Journal of Cultural Heritage, 16*, 753–758.

Sasso, S. (2021). *The tattoo industry is changing – And queer-owned spaces are leading the charge*. PopSugar. https://www.popsugar.com/beauty/queer-tattoo-artists-changing-industry-stereotypes-48374930

Schade, A. (2022). In Bushwick's basement tattoo scene, queer kinship thrives. *Paper Magazine*. https://www.papermag.com/bushwick-basement-tattoo-scene-queer-2658498306.html#rebelltitem24

Schildkrout, E. (2004). Inscribing the body. *Annual Review of Anthropology, 33*(1), 319–344.

Shils, E. (1981). *Tradition*. University of Chicago Press.

Shilling, C. (1991). Educating the body: Physical capital and the production of social inequalities. *Sociology, 25*(4), 653–672.

Shilling, C. (1993). *The body and social theory*. Sage.

Skeggs, B. (1997). *Formations of class and gender*. Sage.

Snape, A. (2020). *I definitely have experienced racism within tattooing*. Things & Ink: Embracing Female Tattoo Culture. http://www.th-ink.co.uk/2020/08/20/i-have-definitely-experienced-racism-within-tattooing/

Spivak, G. C. (1988). Can the Subaltern Speak? In C. Nelson & L. Grossberg (Eds.), *Marxism and the Interpretation of Culture* (pp. 271–313). Macmillan.

Stirn, A., & Hinz, A. (2008). Tattoos, body piercings, and self-injury: Is there a connection? Investigations on a core group of participants practicing body modification. *Psychotherapy Research, 18*(3), 326–333.

Stirn, A., Oddo, S., Peregrinova, L., Philipp, S., & Hinz, A. (2011). Motivations for body piercings and tattoos—The role of sexual abuse and the frequency of body modifications. *Psychiatry Research, 190*, 359–363.

Strohecker, D. P. (2011). The popularization of tattooing: Subcultural resistance and commodification. MA thesis. Department of Sociology, University of Maryland, College Park, MD.

Sullivan, N. (2001). *Tattooed bodies – subjectivity, textuality, ethics and pleasure*. Praeger.

Swami, V., Stieger, S., Pietschnig, J., Voracek, M., Furnham, A., & Tovée, M. J. (2012). The influence of facial piercings and observer personality on perceptions of physical attractiveness and intelligence. *European Psychologist, 17*, 213–221.

Thompson, B. Y. (2015). *Covered in Ink: Tattoos, Women and the Politics of the Body*. NYU Press.

Thorne, G. (2021). Tann Parker is redefining tattooing for dark skin, one Instagram post at a time. *Allure Magazine*. https://www.allure.com/story/tann-parker-ink-the-diaspora-interview0

Torgovnick, M. (1990). *Gone primitive: savage intellects, modern lives*. University of Chicago Press.

Vale, V., & Juno, A. (1989). *Modern primitives*. RE/Search Publications.

Wacquant, L. (2014). *Homines in extremis*: What fighting scholars teach us about habitus. *Body & Society, 20*(2), 3–17.

Walker, K. (2021). *Tattooing guide for darker skin tones*. Liquid Amber Tattoo & Art Collective. https://www.liquidambertattoo.com/blog/2020/9/10/tattooing-guide-for-darker-skin-tones

Weiler, S. M., Tetzlaff, B.-O., Herzberg, P. Y., & Jacobsen, T. (2021). When personality gets under the skin: Need for uniqueness and body modifications. *PLoS ONE, 16*(3), e0245158. https://doi.org/10.1371/journal.pone.0245158

Westerfield, H. V., Stafford, A. B., Speroni, K. G., & Daniel, M. G. (2012). Patients' perceptions of patient care providers with tattoos and/or body piercings. *Journal of Nursing Administration, 42*, 160–164. https://doi.org/10.1097/NNA.0b013e31824809d6

Wohlrab, S., Stahl, J., & Kappeler, P. M. (2007). Modifying the body: Motivations for getting tattooed and pierced. *Body Image*, 4(1), 87–95. https://doi.org/10.1016/j.bodyim.2006.12.001

Wolf, N. (1991). *The beauty myth*. Chatto and Windus.

INDEX

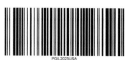